DISCLAIMER

LifeVantage® and its Affiliates DO NOT claim to cure, heal, prevent, mitigate or diagnose any disease.

This information is for educational purposes only.

LifeVantage® Consultants are independent contractors and are not employees. Any views and statements expressed or implied do not necessarily reflect the views of LifeVantage.

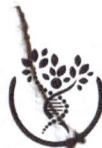

ACTIVATE
WELLNESS

Where it all started

It all began back in the lab with the discovery and perfection of Protandim Nrf2 by award winning scientists. Protandim Nrf2 became famous overnight, when it caught the attention of an ABC news reporting company who featured it in an all-positive news segment.

Three things came from this news report:

1. The results were astounding! John Quinones, the news reporter, used himself as a test subject and saw a reduction of oxidative stress by 45% in less than two weeks.
2. Scientists and Researchers were blown away with the results and reached out to the company to begin conducting their own studies on Protandim Nrf2. To date, more than 40 universities have funded their own studies on Protandim Nrf2 and more than 30 Peer Reviewed studies (Gold Standard Research) have been published, validating its effectiveness.
3. People wanted and needed Protandim!

As it was a small biotech company at the time, it took several months to fulfil these orders before it was placed on the shelves in nutrition stores. However, as people were unaware of terms such as 'Oxidative Stress' and 'Nrf2 Activation', marketing was a challenge.

Our success wasn't due to fancy packaging or expensive marketing – it was because our customers loved their results and couldn't help but to tell others about their experience. So, if our customers' success stories were fueling our own, why not pay them for it? LifeVantage made a bold choice – pulling the successful products off the shelves and creating an opportunity for any customer to earn money by becoming a LifeVantage Consultant.

Since the discovery and success of Protandim Nrf2, LifeVantage has continued to pour funding into research and development to further support the body through activation. Our latest breakthrough is with TrueScience Liquid Collagen. The world's FIRST Activating Collagen that works in synergy with Protandim Nrf2 to increase collagen density 100%!

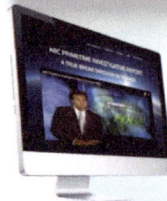

To view the ABC Report which aired in 2005 **Scan Here**

Ready, Set, Glow!

Radiant, youthful skin emanates from within as the result of combining two products boasting exquisitely timeless advantages. The patented synergy of TrueScience® Liquid Collagen and Protandim® Nrf2 Synergizer® works harmoniously to restore collagen from within and safeguard the well-being of your skin while addressing the root cause of aging within your cells.

TrueScience® Liquid Collagen uniquely activates your body's ability to produce collagen to help reduce the appearance of fine lines and wrinkles and improve moisture and texture.

Protandim® Nrf2 Synergizer® activates the cellular pathway responsible for antioxidant production, reducing oxidative stress by 40% in the first 30 days winding back the cellular clock.

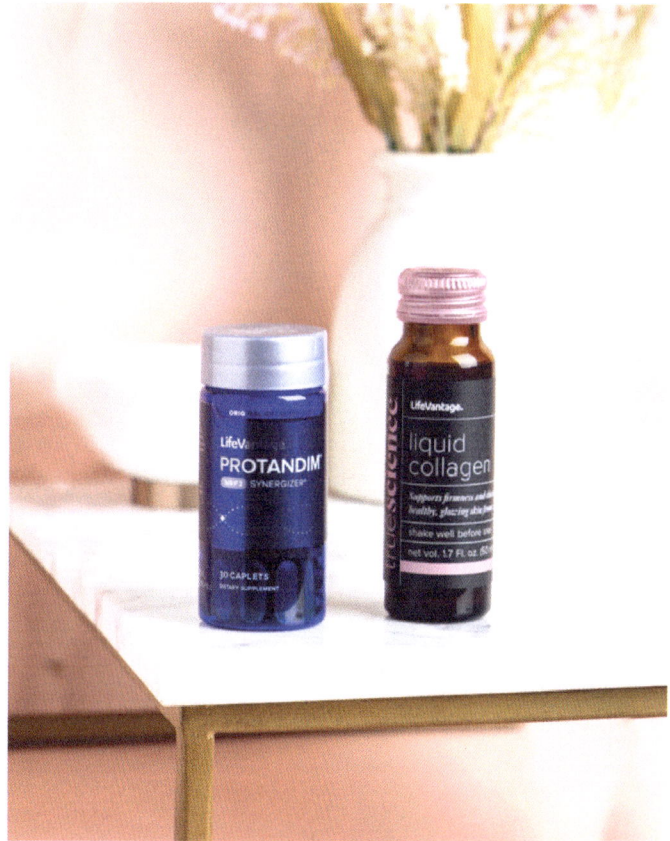

The combination of TrueScience® Liquid Collagen and Protandim® Nrf2 Synergizer® are proven to increase collagen production 100% and support the body's natural stress response.

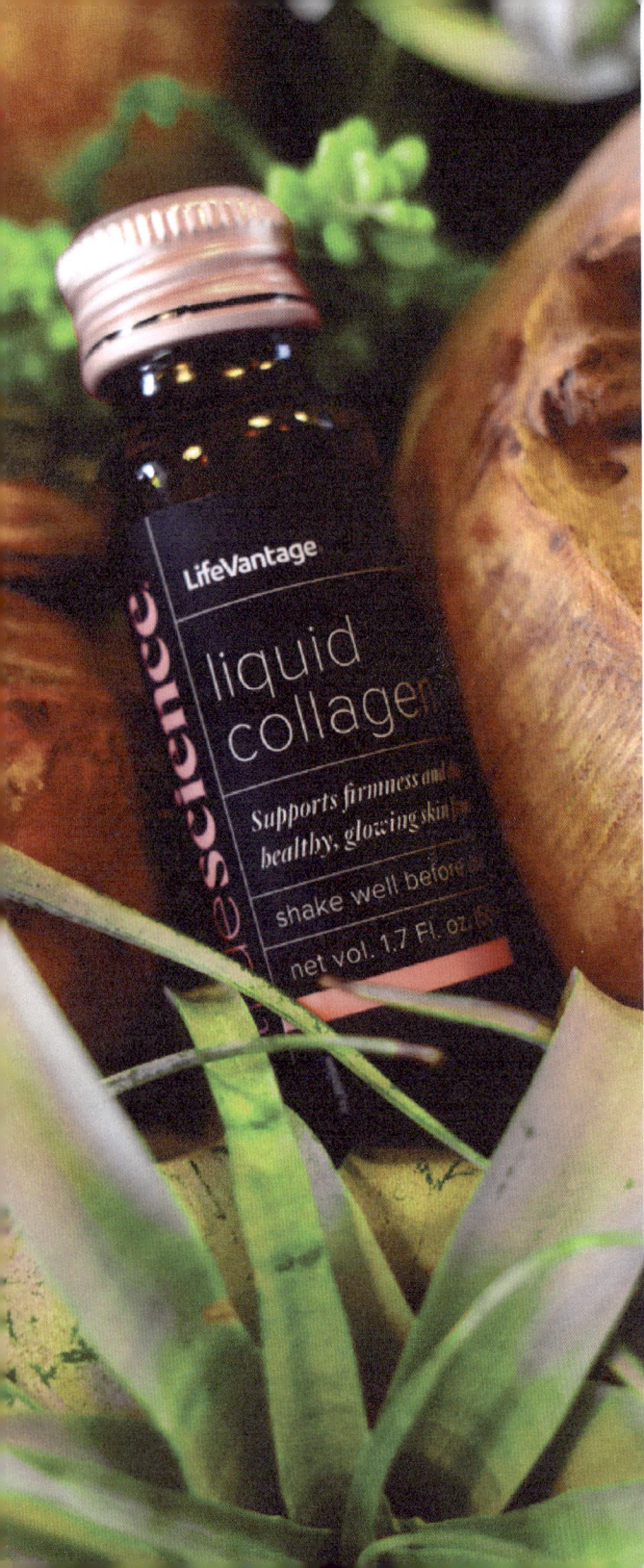

TrueScience® Liquid Collagen

activate.
replenish.
maintain. *

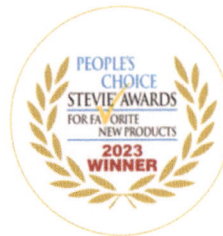
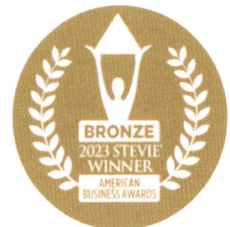

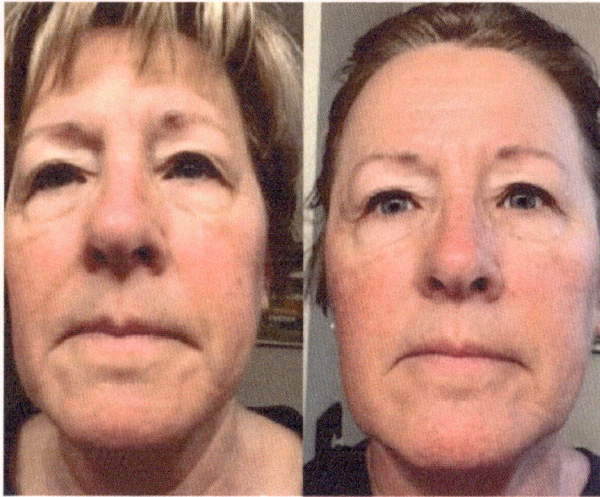

Day 1 **Day 15**

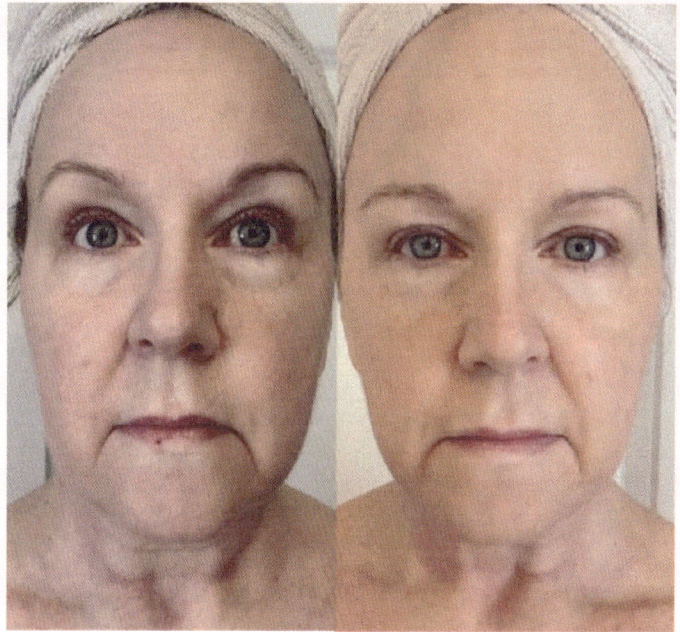

Day 1 **Day 365**

On a premium liquid marine collagen for over 2 years and didn't expect this much change!!!

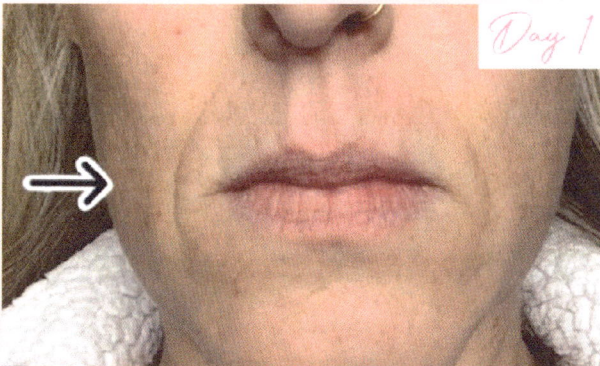

Day 1

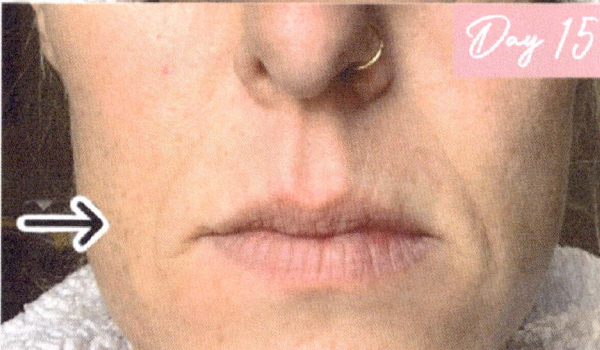

Day 15

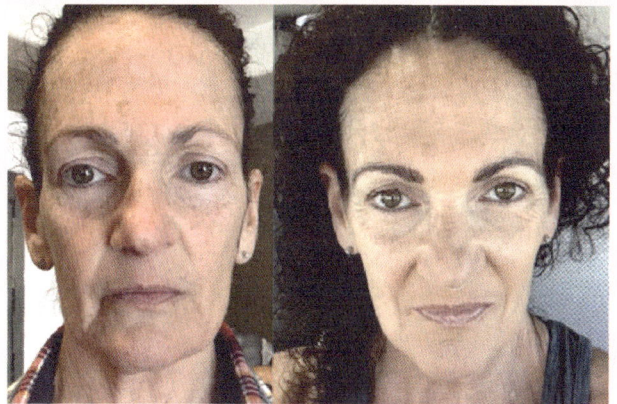

Day 1 **4 Months**

Individual results may vary.

Why Collagen?

Collagen in a structural protein that makes up about 25%-35% of all the proteins in your body. The body produces collagen proteins from the amino acids that you take in through food.

This process starts to steeply decline around the age of 30, leading to a large reduction in collagen density which then causes **saggy, dull and wrinkled looking skin.**

Before

8 Months

TrueScience Liquid Collagen

We are the only formula on the market that approaches skin and collagen health 3 different ways:

1.ACTIVATE the genes responsible for collagen production so that the body begins producing more collagen.

2.REPLENISH the collagen that has been lost (the typical approach in the market).

3.MAINTAIN by slowing and minimizing the existing collagen in your body from breaking down.

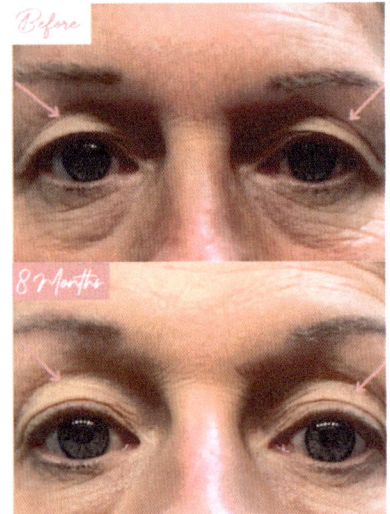

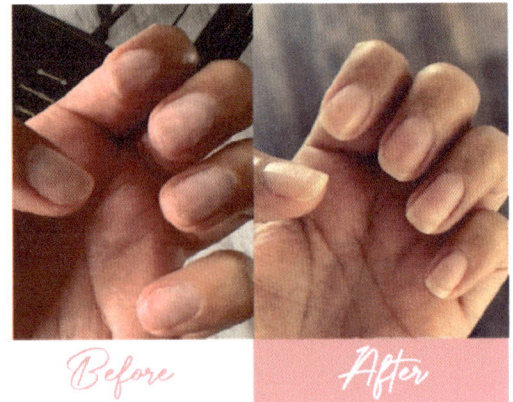

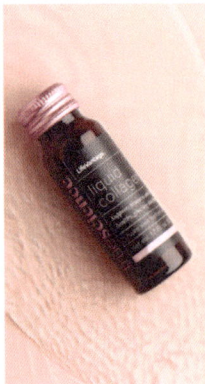

Before   After

What does it do?

provides antioxidants

helps reduce joint pain associated with osteoarthritis

source of the non-essential amino acids (alanine, arginine, aspartic acid, glutamic acid, glycine, proline, serine, tyrosine) involved in collagen protein synthesis.

source of essential amino acid (histidine, isoleucine, leucine, lysine, methionine, phenylalanine, threonine, valine) for the maintenance of good health (and involved in collagen protein synthesis)

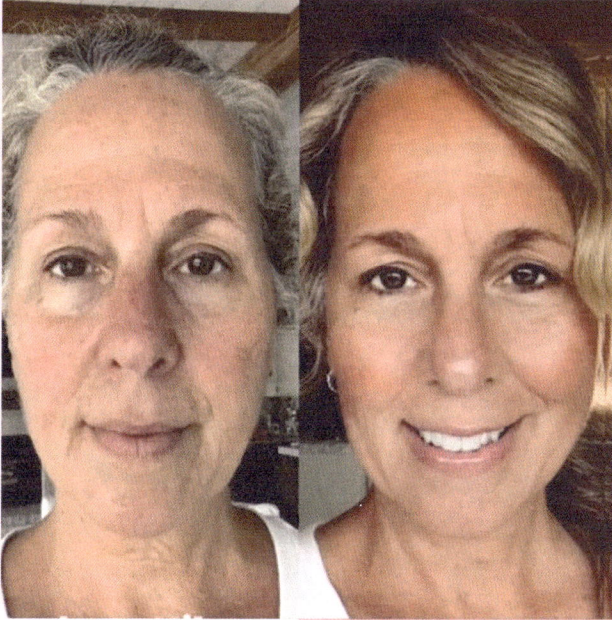

Before · *1 year*

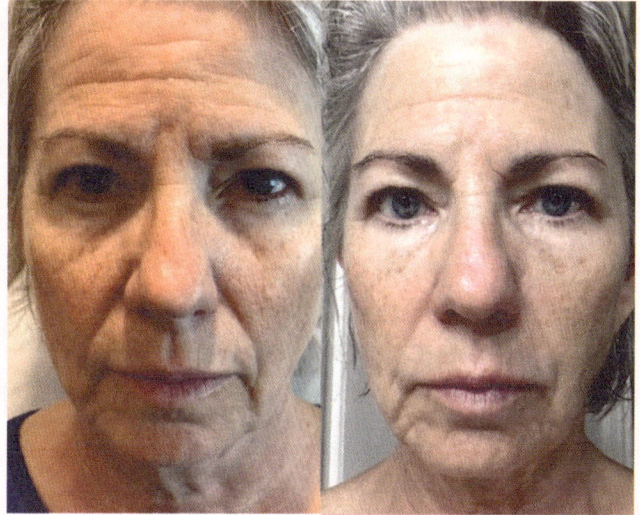

Day 1 · *Day 365*

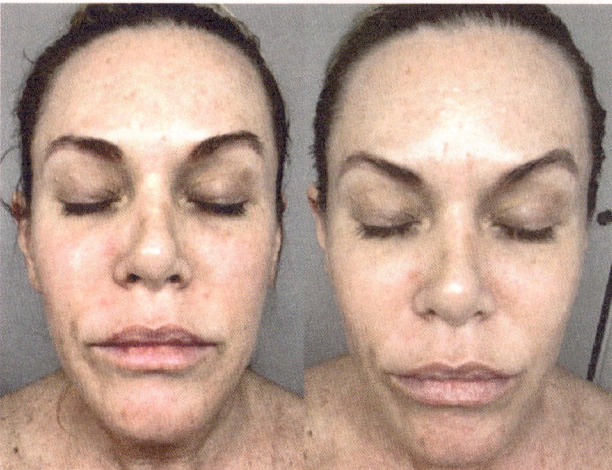

Before · *After*

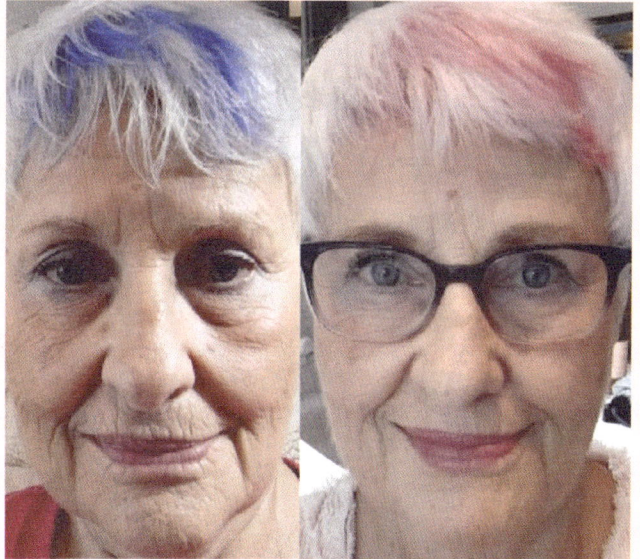

Before · *After*

Individual results may vary.

What's in it?

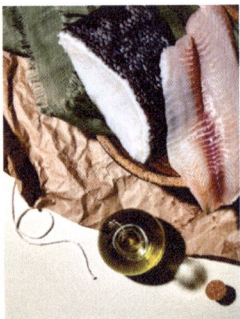

Fish Collagen Peptides

5,000mg of hydrolyzed marine peptides from responsibly and sustainably caught fish.

These 10 types of collagen peptides provide amino acids to support collagen density, skin elasticity, and skin moisture for a youthful appearance.*

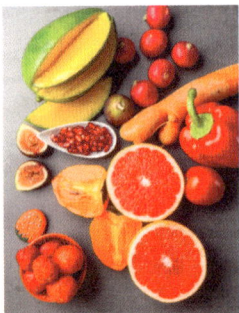

Lycopene Beadlets

A carotenoid antioxidant that supports the collagen network throughout the body. This natural concentrate derived from red, orange and pink fruits, provides many essential antioxidants which help the body fight against oxidative stress.

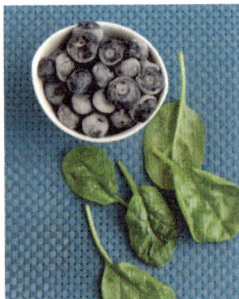

Berry and Spinach Extracts

Blueberry powder (vaccinium augustifolia), Acerola Berry extract (malpighia emarginata), and Spinach Juice Powder (spinacia oleracea). Our blend of blueberry powder, acerola berry and spinach juice extract supplies vitamin C and antioxidants.

True Science. True Results.

Results based on 8-week clinical trial on key ingredients in Liquid Collagen. Individual results may vary.

COLLAGEN DENSITY INCREASED BY 42%*

DEPTH OF CROWS FEET REDUCED BY 22%*

SKIN ELASTICITY INCREASED BY 8%*

SKIN ROUGHNESS REDUCED BY 10%*

BLOOD CATALASE (CAT) ANTIOXIDANT LEVEL INCREASED BY 202%*

what's not in it

No added sugar	Non-GMO	Gluten free
No artificial sweeteners	Dairy free	Soy free

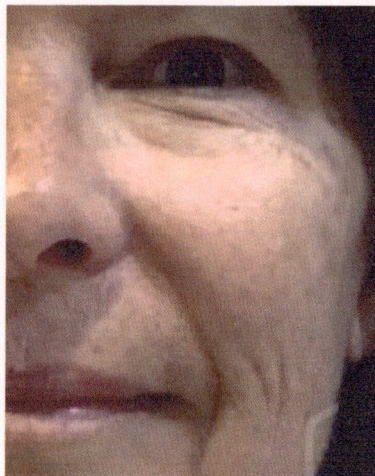 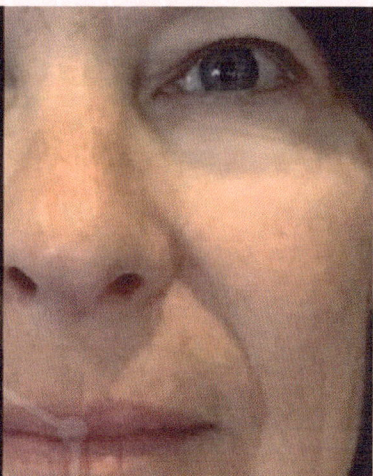 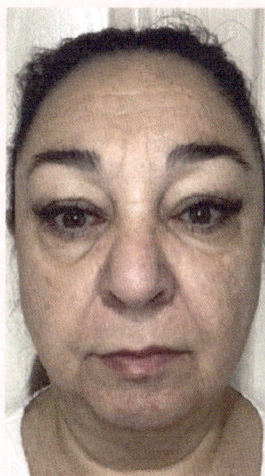 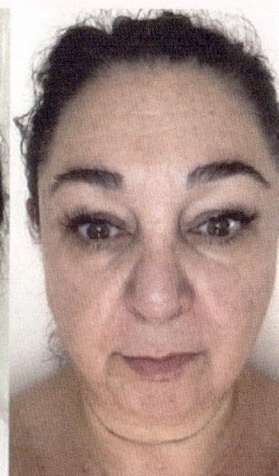

Day 1 **Day 15** **Day 1** **Day 10**

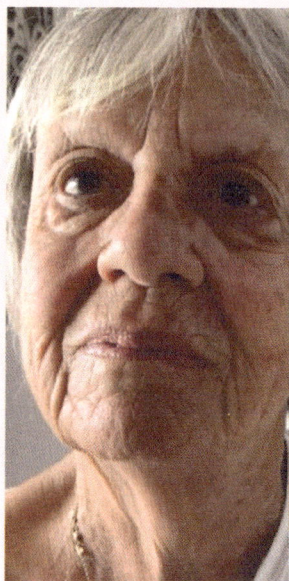 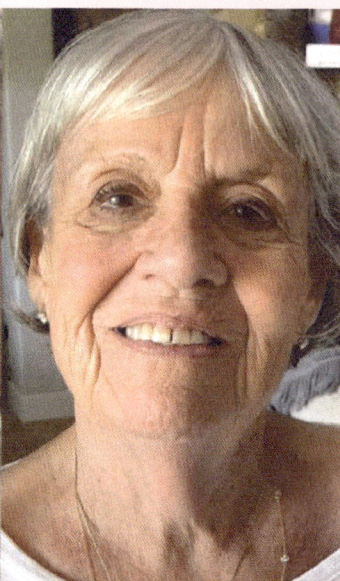 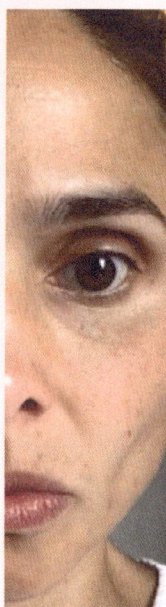 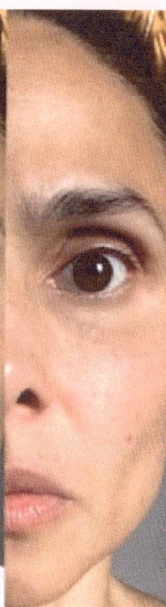 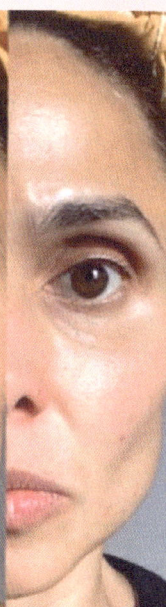 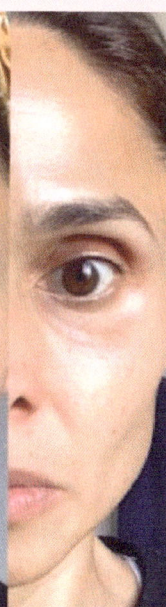

Day 1 **Day 75** **Day 1** **Day 30** **Day 45** **Day 60**

Individual results may vary.

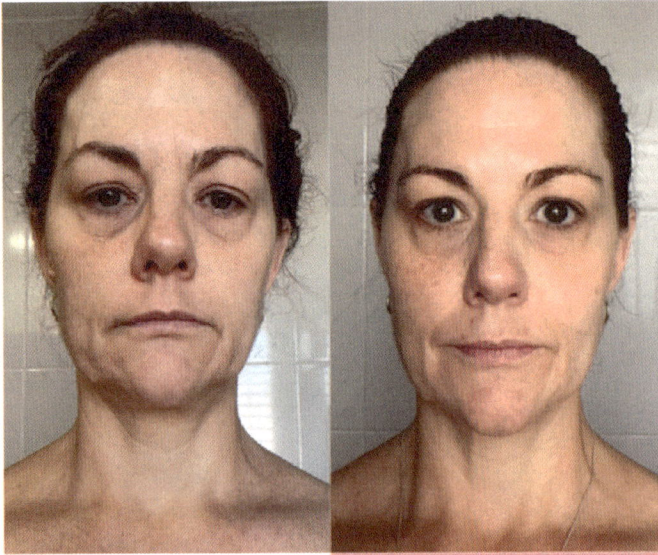

Day 1   Day 40

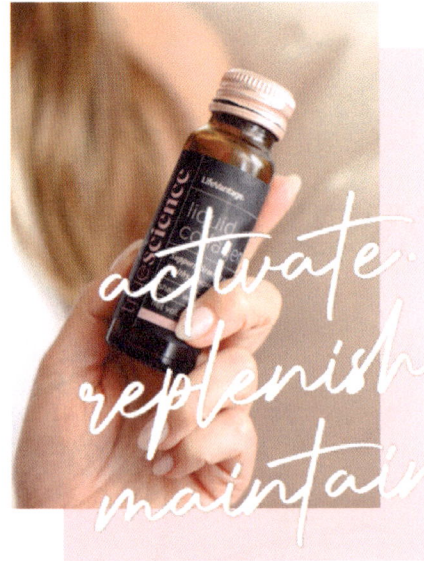

activate.
replenish
maintain

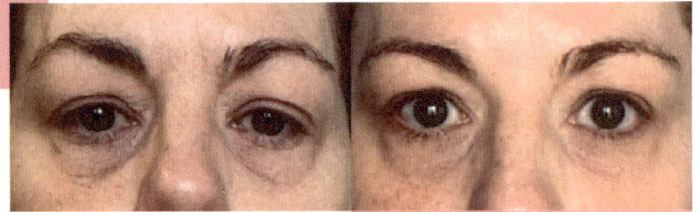

Before   Day 40

Why Liquid?

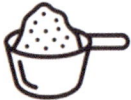

powder
10-30% absorption

Large collagen protein pieces are hard to digest. they need to be broken down by enzymes.

TrueScience liquid collagen uses hydrolyzed collagen, chopped up into smaller pieces, so your body doesn't have to break them down.

liquid
90%+ absorption

Hydrolyzed collagen pieces are highly water-soluble whereas regular collagen is not, so the most efficient form is a liquid. This creates extremely high bioavailability.

Individual results may vary.

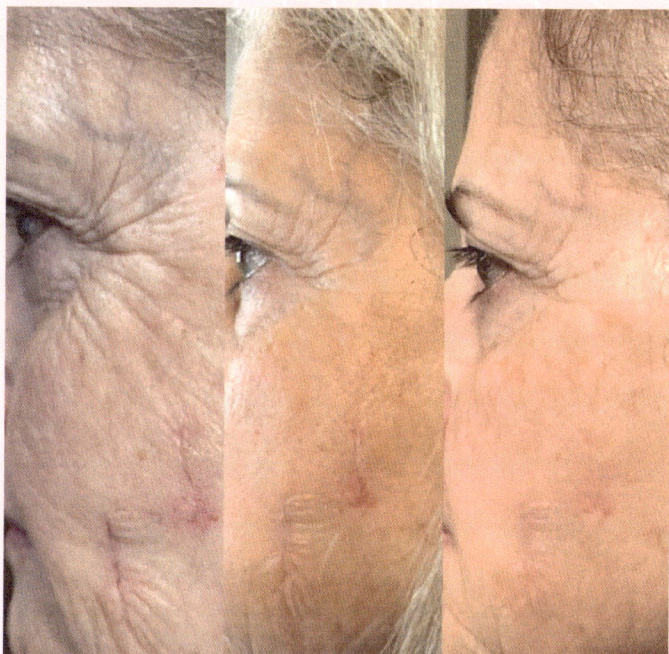

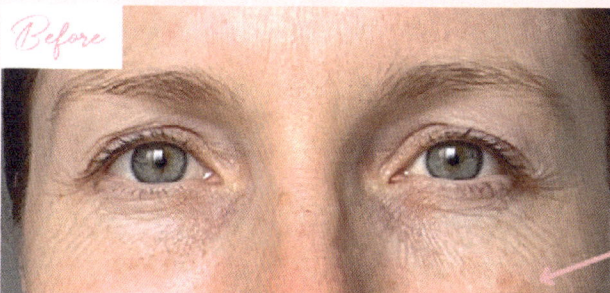

Before

Day 1 **Month 1** **Month 6**

3 Months

6 Months

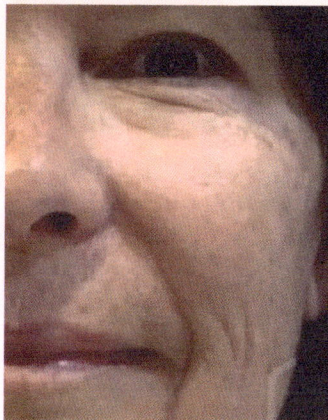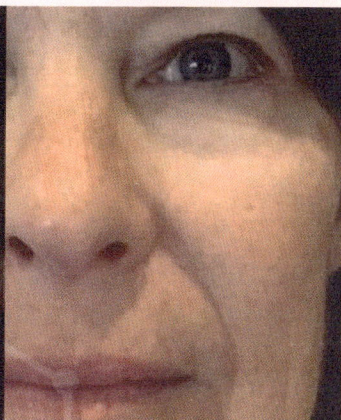

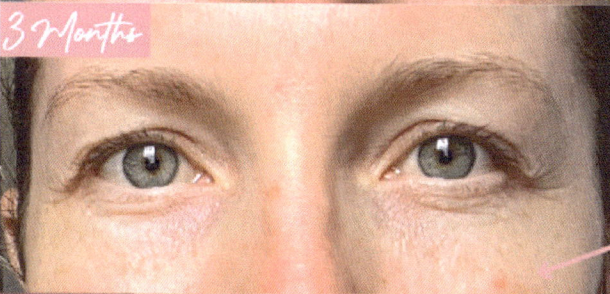

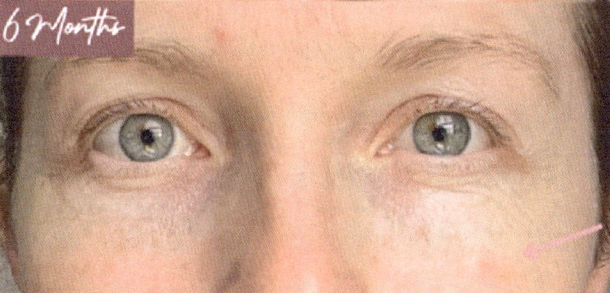

Day 1 **Day 15**

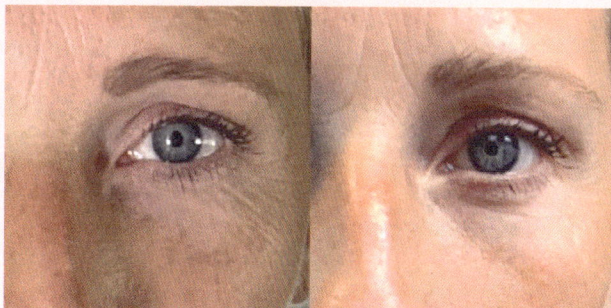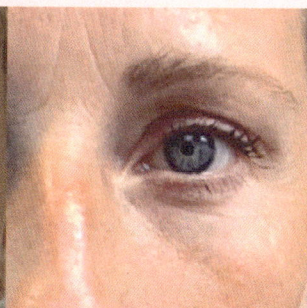

Day 1 **Day 21**

Individual results may vary.

Studies TrueScience® Liquid Collagen

Week 0   Week 4   Week 8

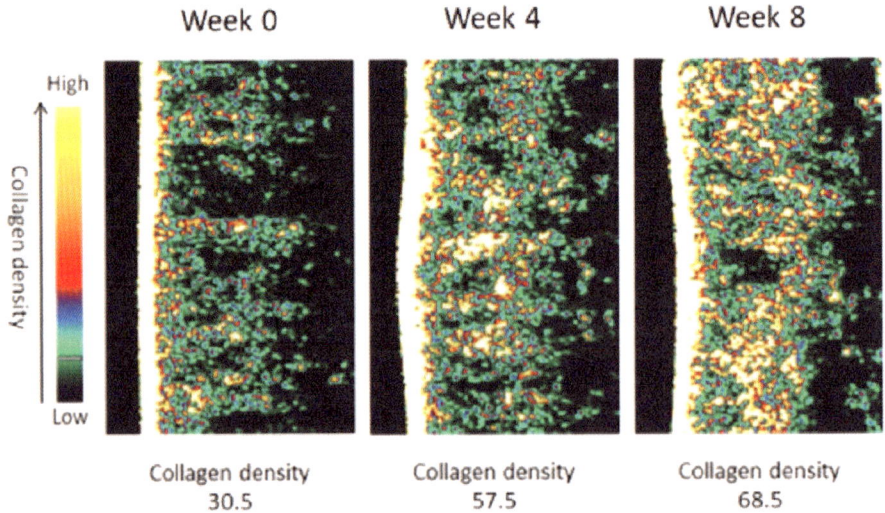

High

Collagen density

Low

*Results based on an 8-week clinical trial on key ingredients in Liquid Collagen. Individual results may vary.

Collagen density
30.5

Collagen density
57.5

Collagen density
68.5

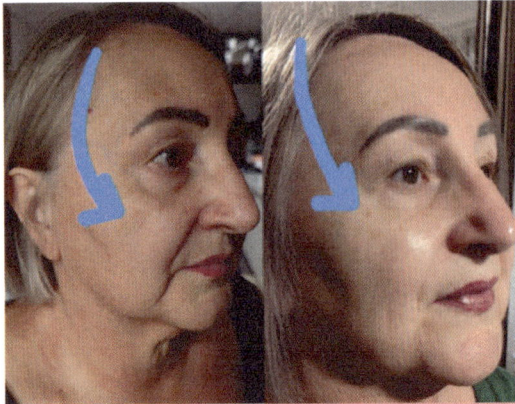

Before

After

| The difference is out of bounds. I can se...
Thank you! Yeah she is beautiful ❤️ she went to a skin aesthetician and was quoted $3000 every 9 months for bio-remodeling to fix the fat loss in her cheeks. The hollows are literally filling out!

Individual results may vary.

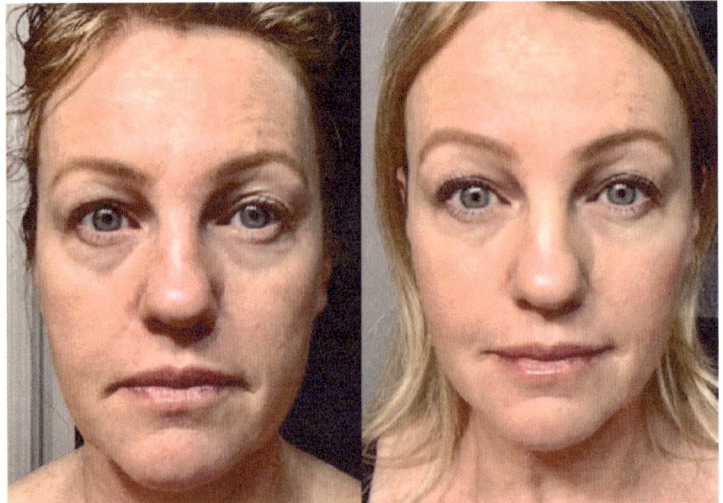

Before

After

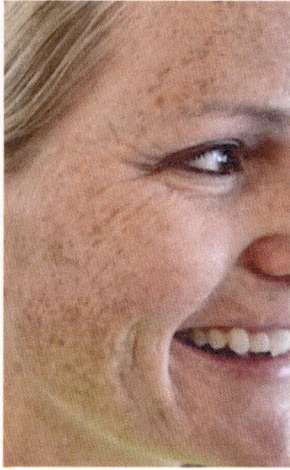
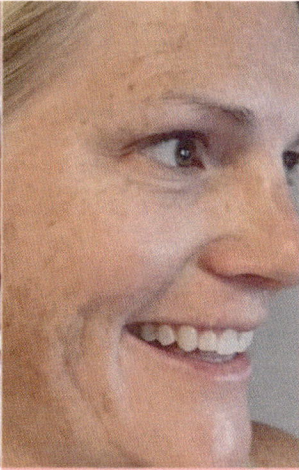
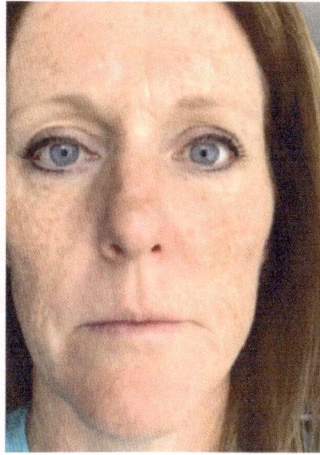
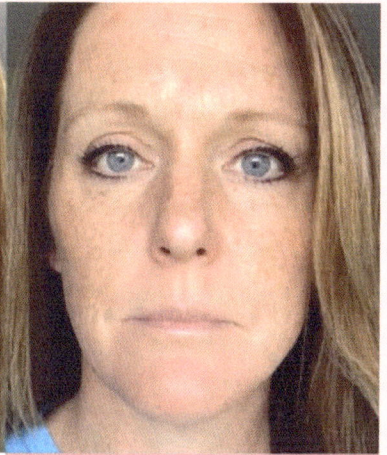

Before *After* *Day 1* *Day 90*

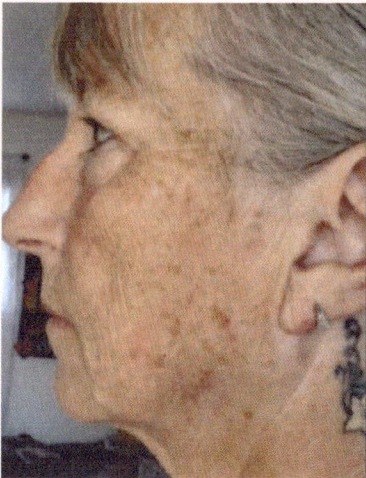
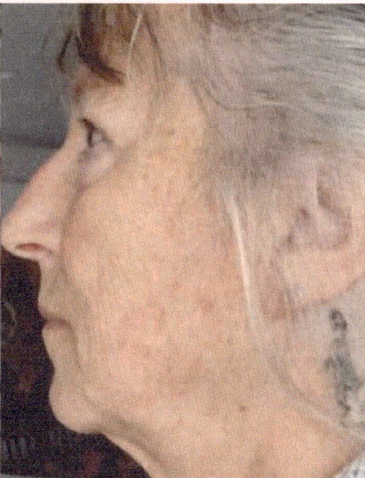
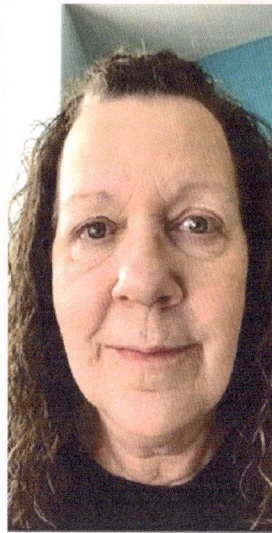
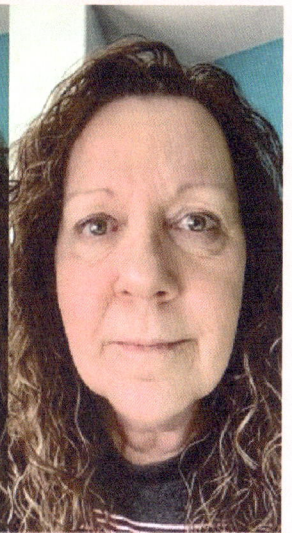

Day 1 *Day 60* *Day 1* *Day 120*

Individual results may vary.

say hello to #trueconfidence

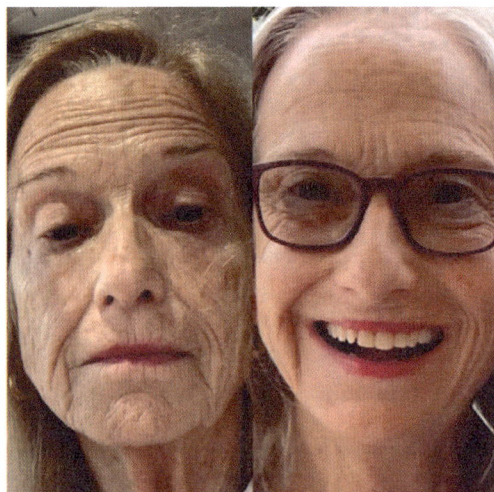

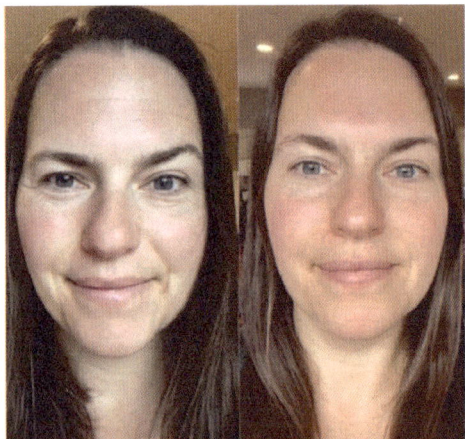

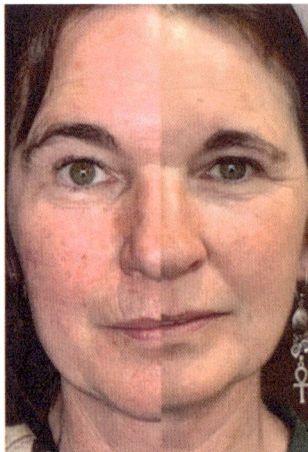

Before *5 Months* *Before* *3 Months*

Before *5 Months*

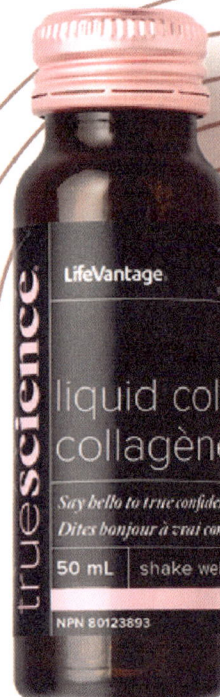

Get glowing, gorgeous skin with a daily boost of collagen and activating botanicals. The proprietary ingredients in this delicious blend have been clinically shown to deliver visible support to skin health and hydration in 8 weeks or less. Your skin looks smoother, softer, and more even, while Liquid Collagen works from within to reduce collagen breakdown and improve skin elasticity.

It also helps protect against the damaging effects of oxidative stress, caused by free radicals. With more youthful-looking skin, you'll glow with True Confidence. You get real results that you can see—and feel.*

Individual results may vary.

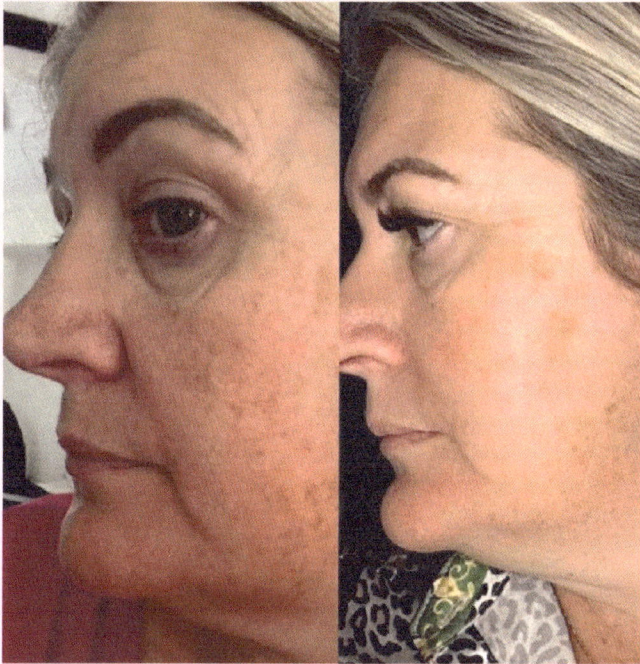

Day 1 **Day 100**

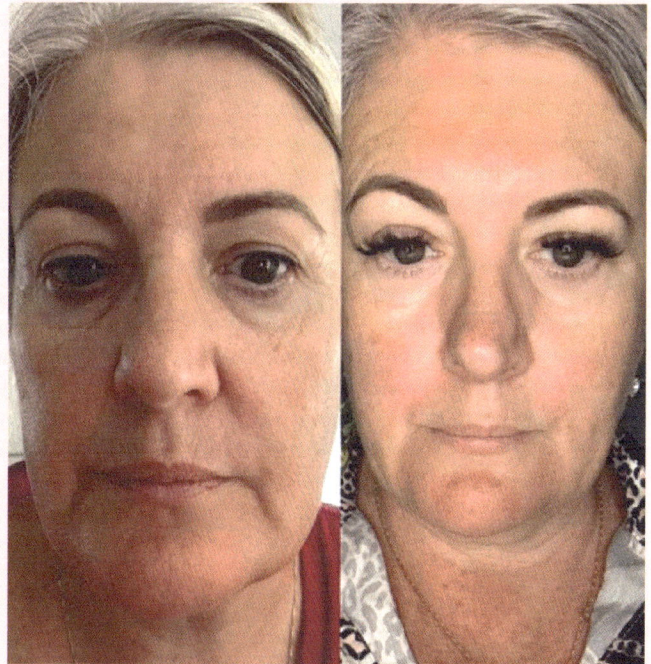

Day 1 **Day 100**

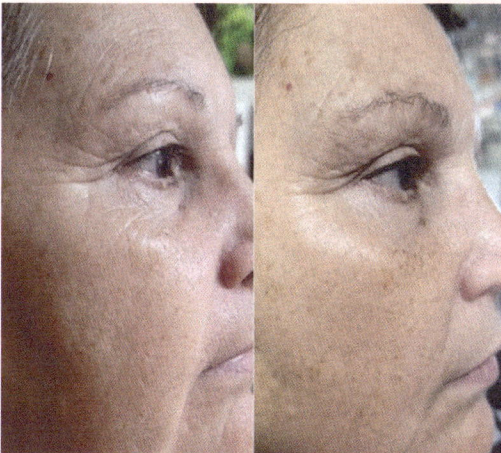

Day 1 **Day 6**

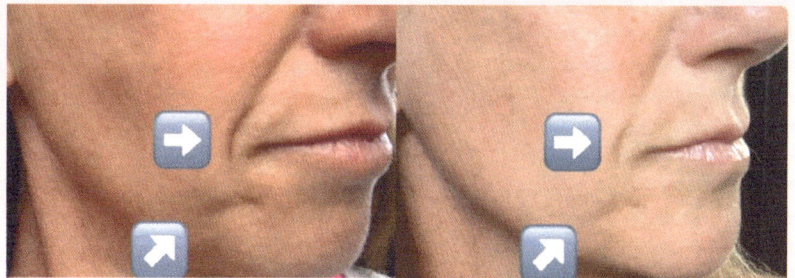

Day 1 **Day 55**

*activate. replenish. maintain.**

Individual results may vary.

Did you know?

There is a difference between taking collagen supplements, and having your body make its own! Making your own is far more effective!
You can now ACTIVATE the pathways in your body, responsible for collagen production AND turn down the genes responsible for collagen breakdown!!

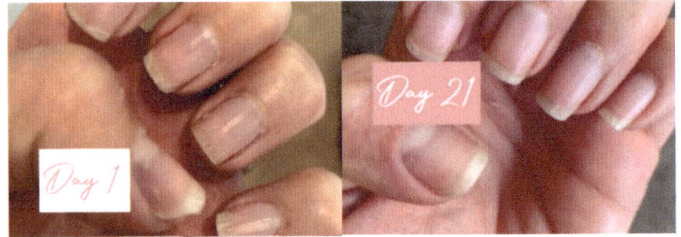

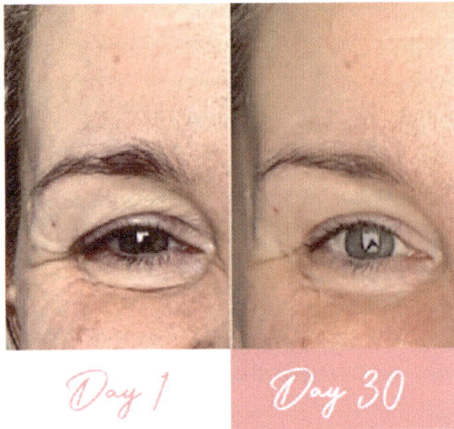

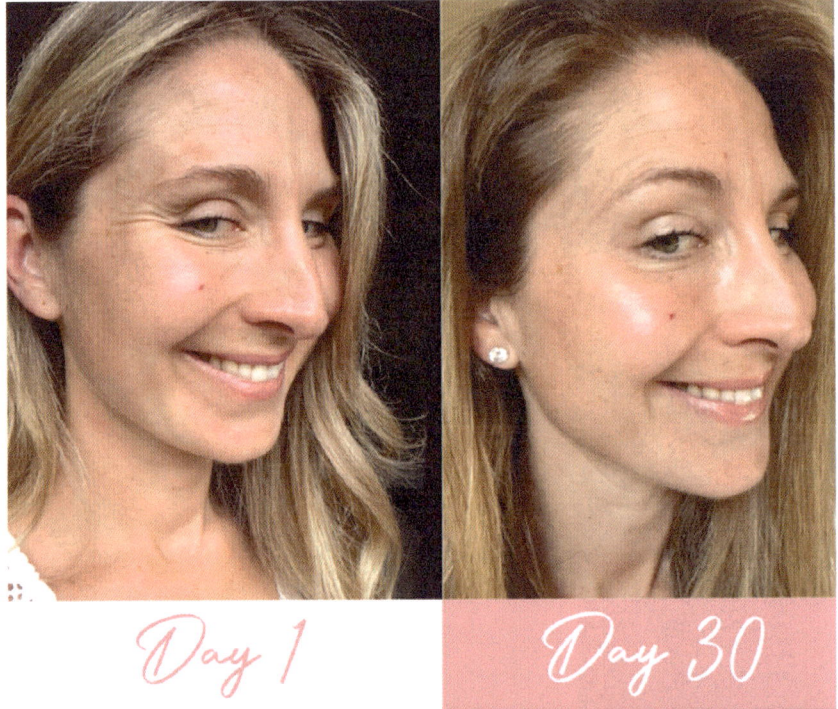

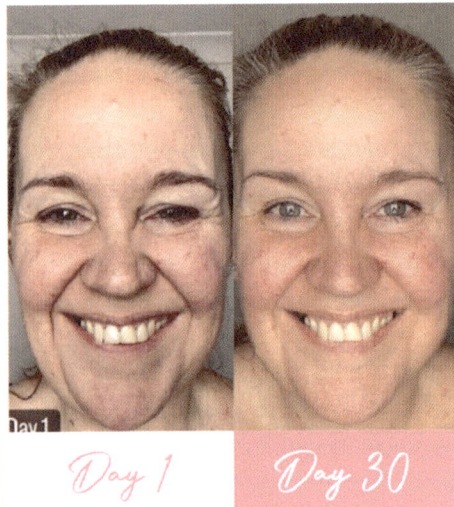

Day 1
Day 21

Day 1
Day 30

Day 1
Day 30

Day 1
Day 30

These are my results in just 30 days from activated liquid collagen and Nrf2 Activation:
- Wrinkles are disappearing
- Finger nails have never been so strong
- Inflammation and pain in my knuckles have gone
- Way more energy
- Better recovery after workouts
- Gut health has improved - I'm not as hungry and cravings have gone

Individual results may vary.

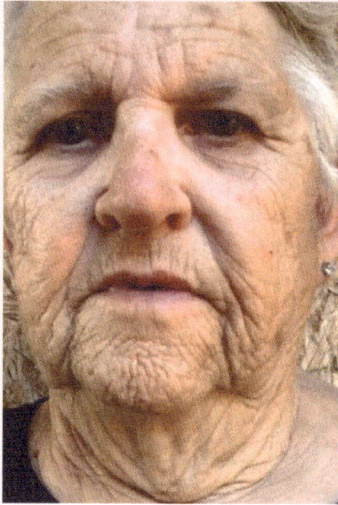
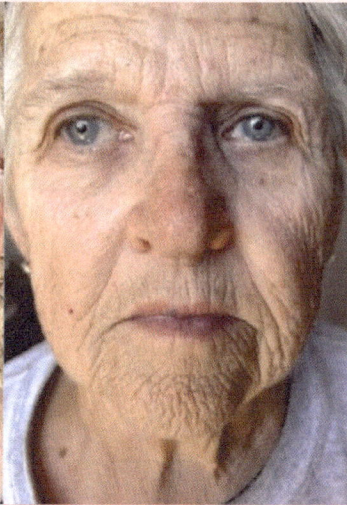
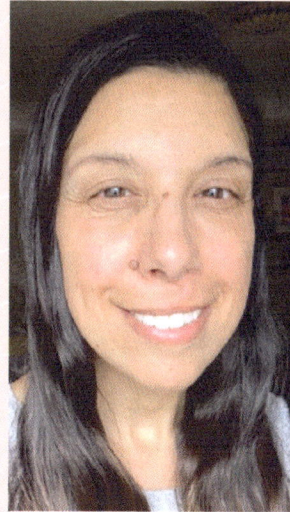
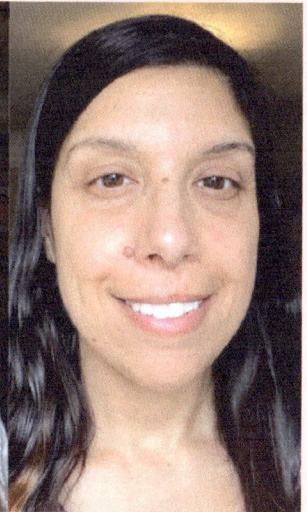

Day 1 **Day 55** *Day 1* **Day 30**

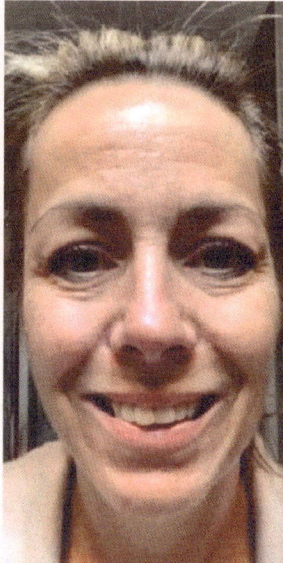
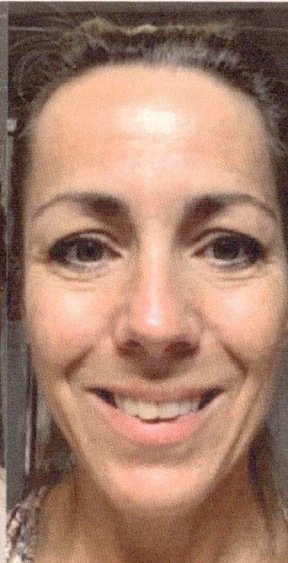
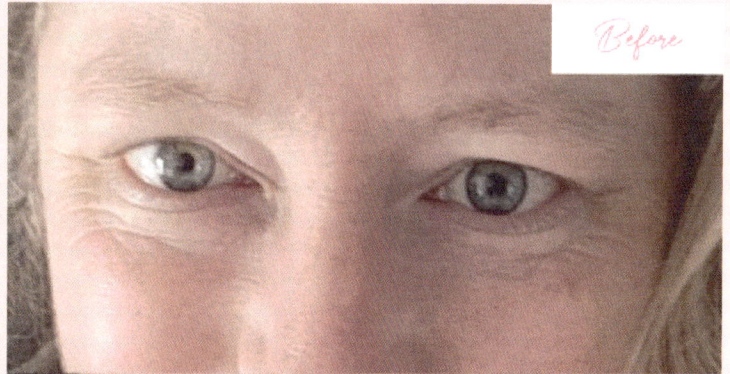

Before

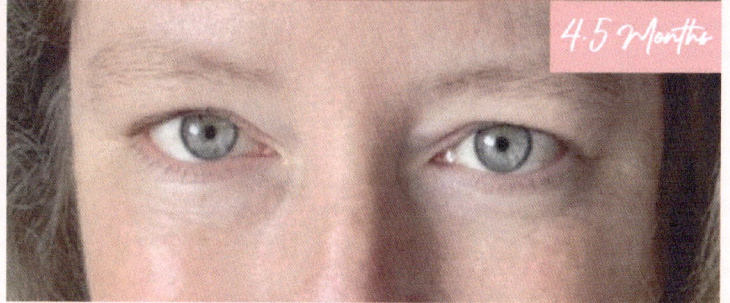

4.5 Months

Day 1 **Day 21**

Individual results may vary.

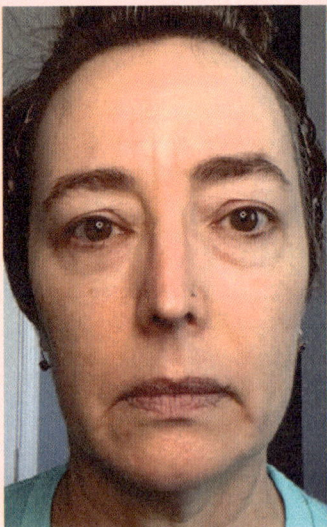
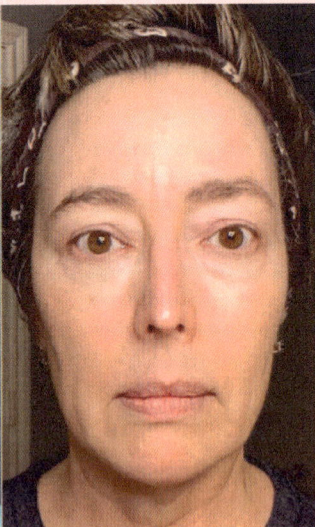
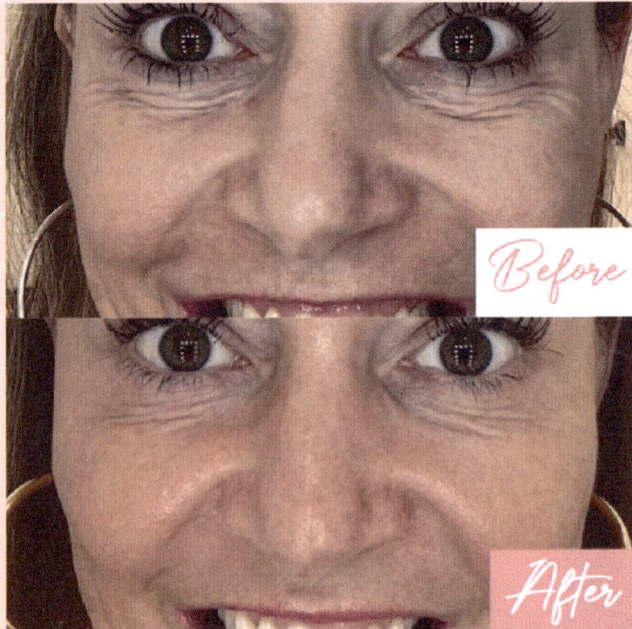

Day 1   **7 Months**

Before

After

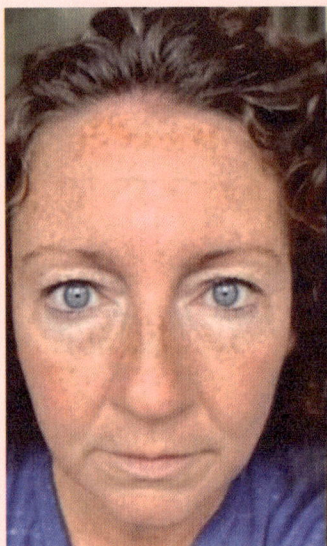
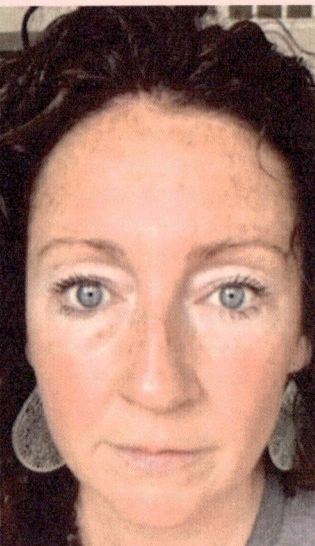
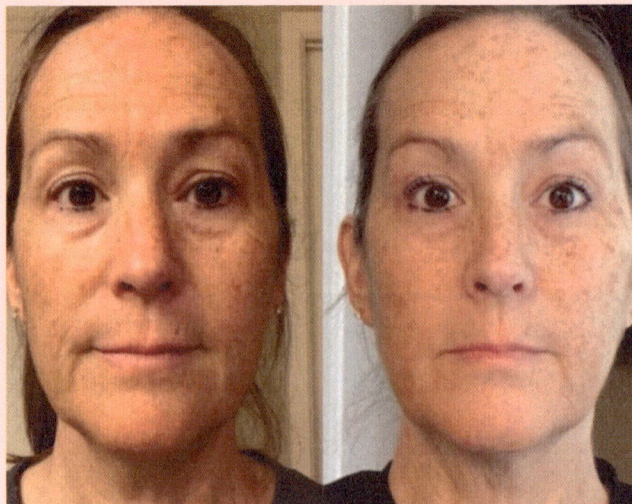

Day 1   **6 Months**

Before   **7 Months**

Individual results may vary.

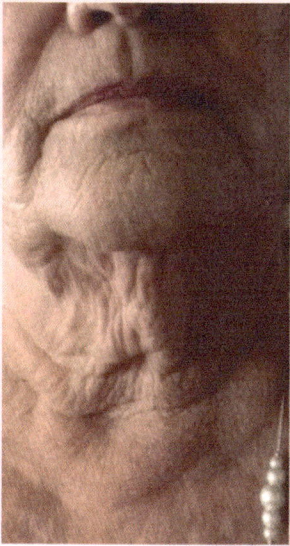
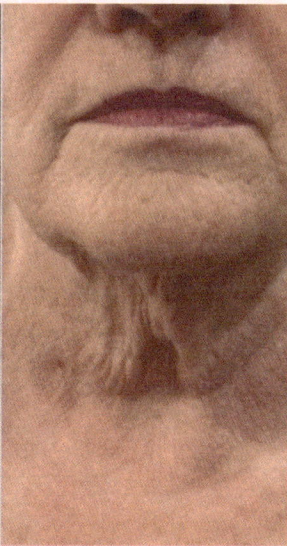
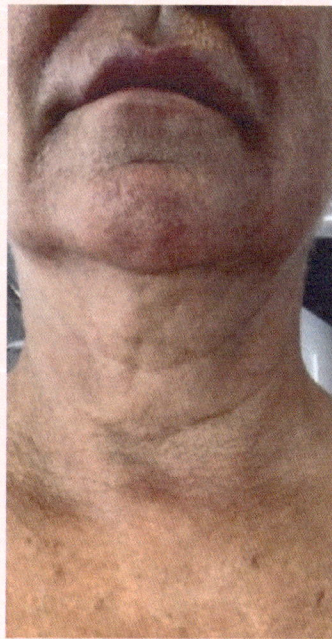
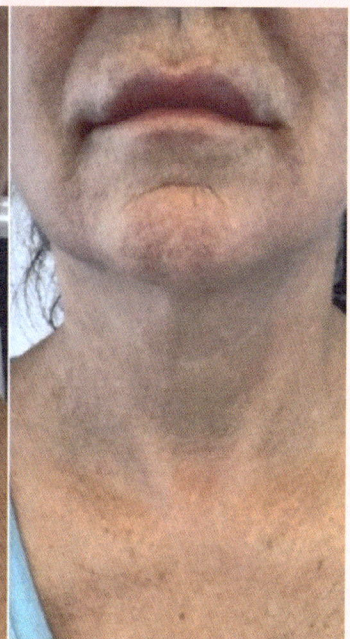

Day 1

Day 45

Day 1

Day 7

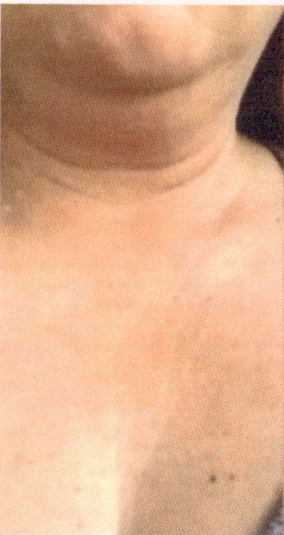
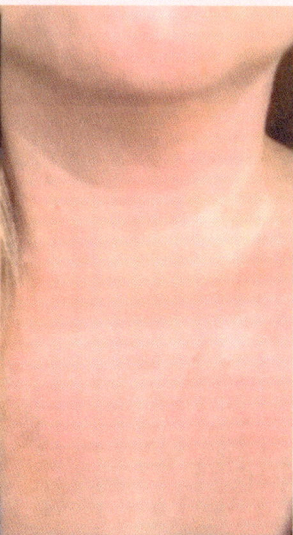
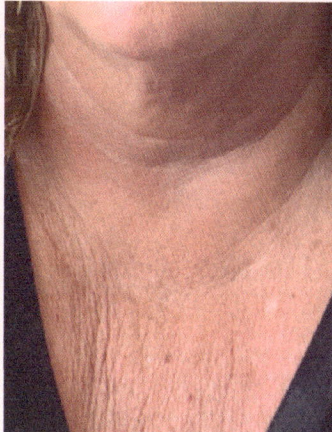
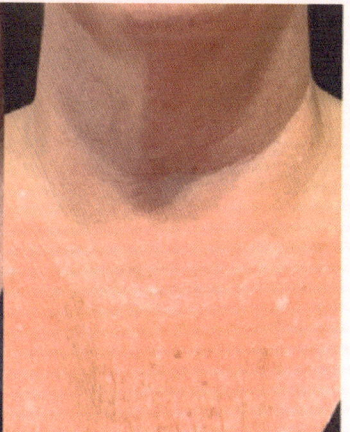

Before

After

Day 1

Day 70

Individual results may vary.

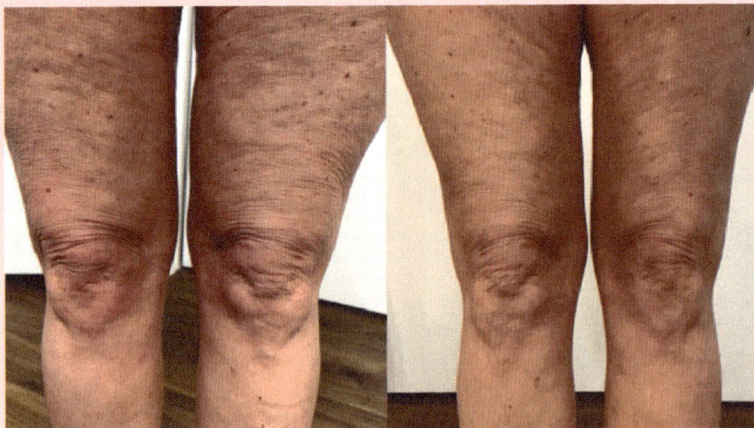

Before — After

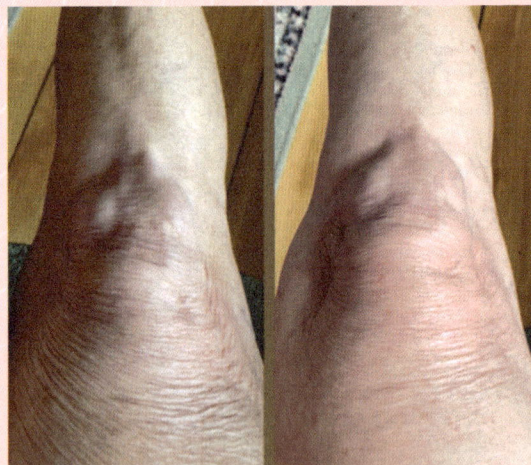

Before — After

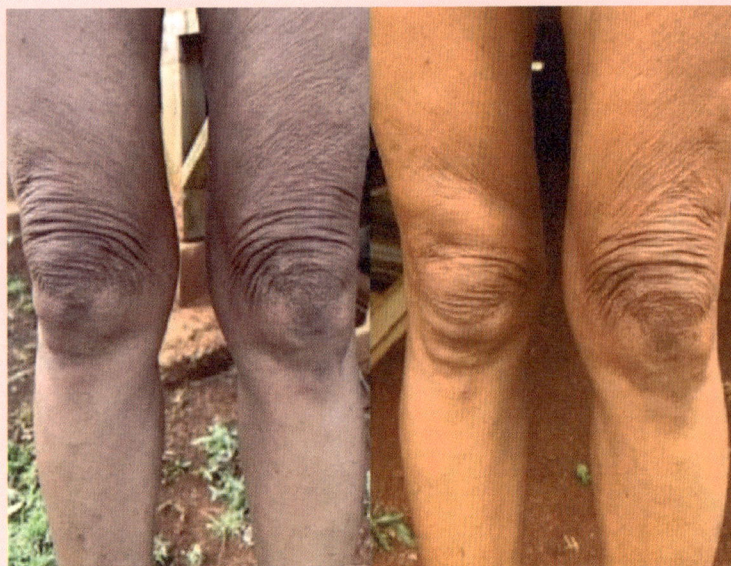

Before — After

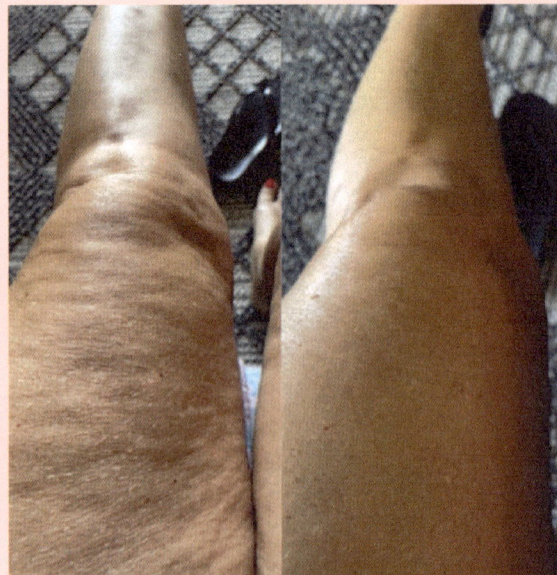

Day 1 — 3 Months

Individual results may vary.

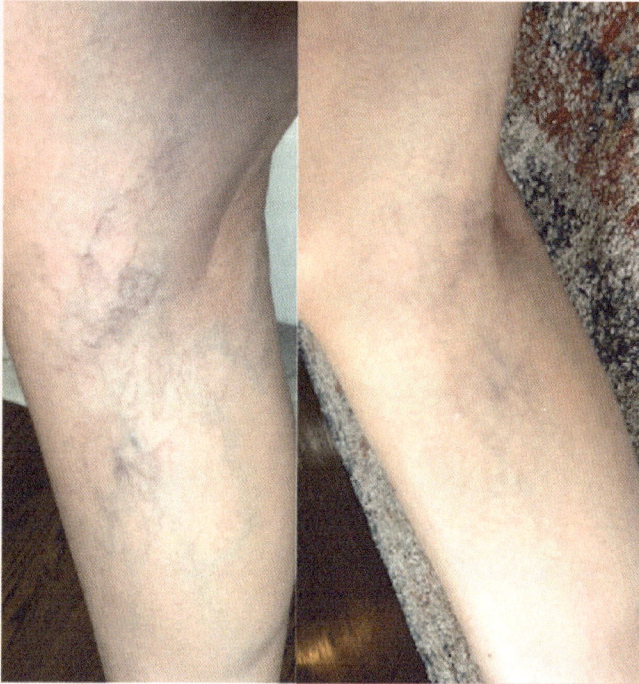
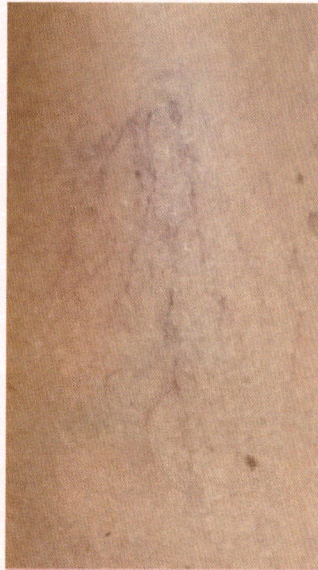

Day 1

5 Months

Day 1

Day 45

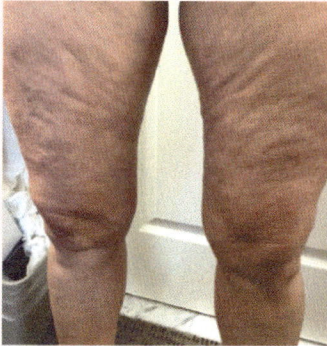
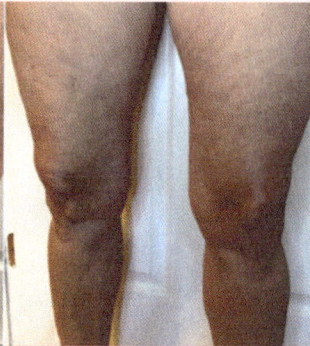
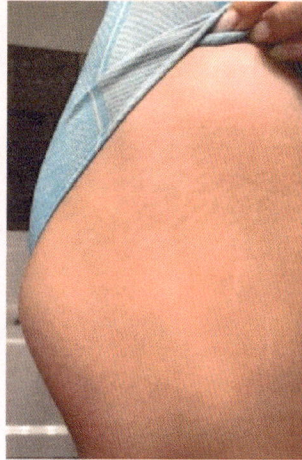
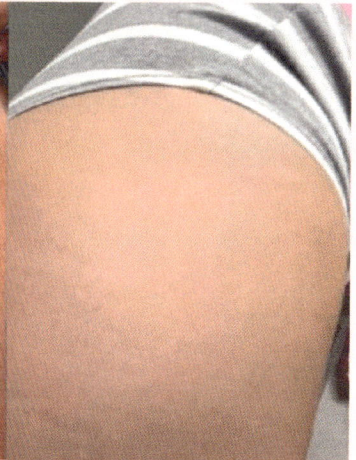

Day 1

Day 14

Day 1

Day 30

Individual results may vary.

Before

After

Day 1

Day 20

8 months

Before

After

Day 1

Day 28

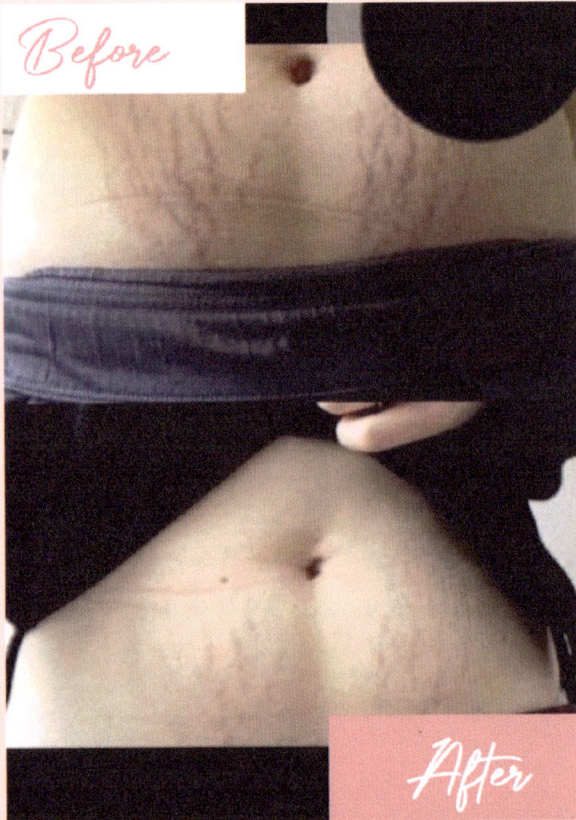

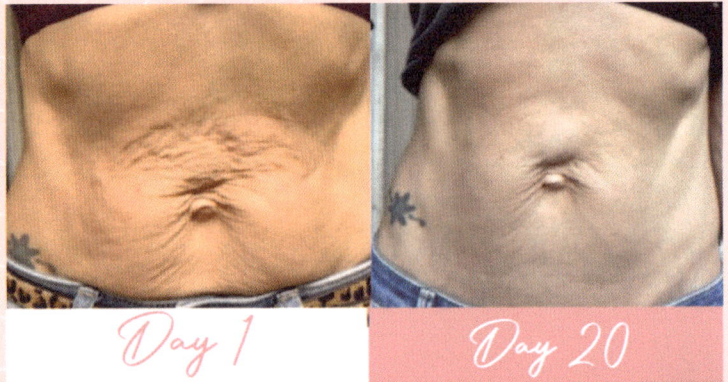

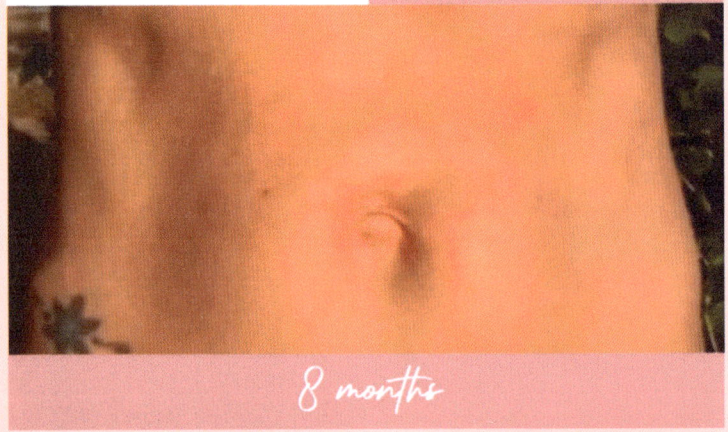

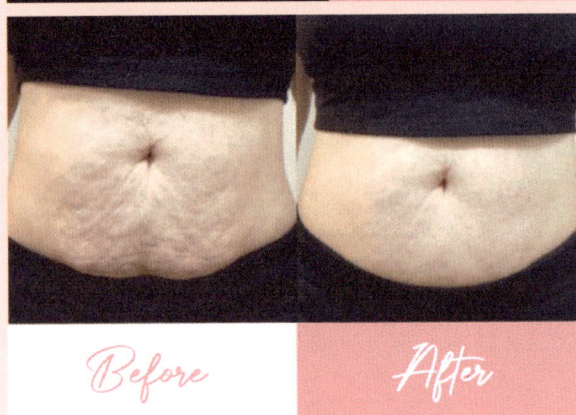

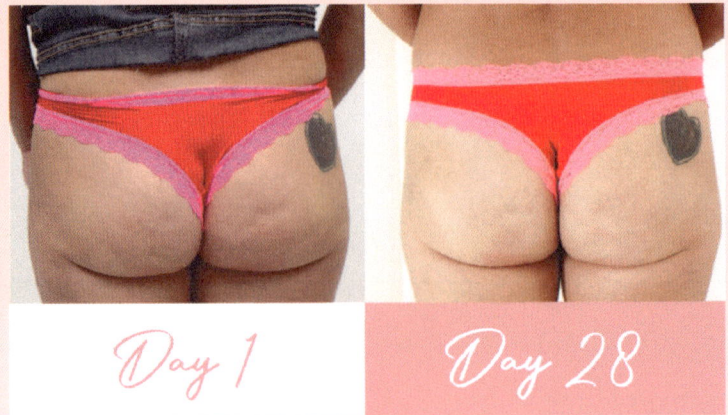

Individual results may vary.

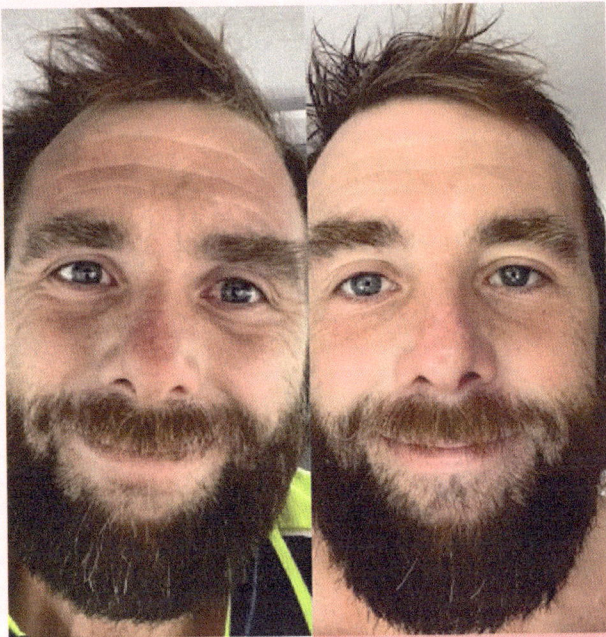

Before

After

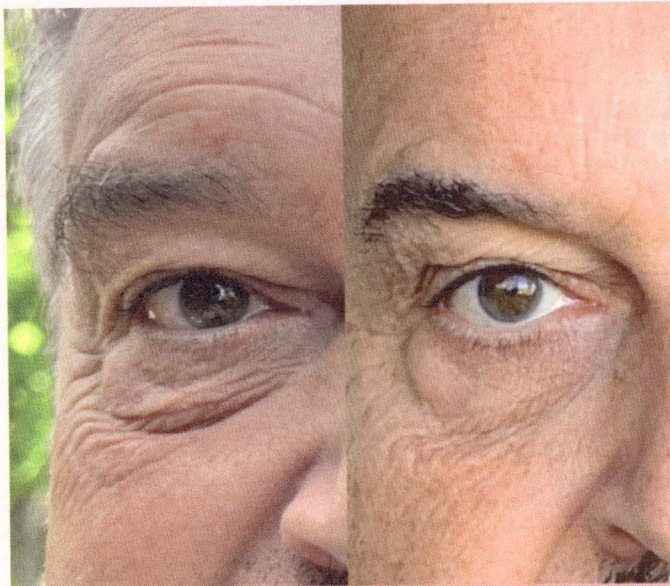

Day 1

Day 180

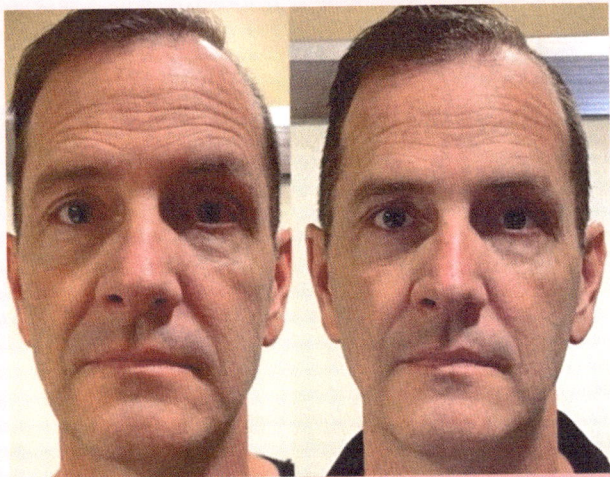

Day 1

Day 90

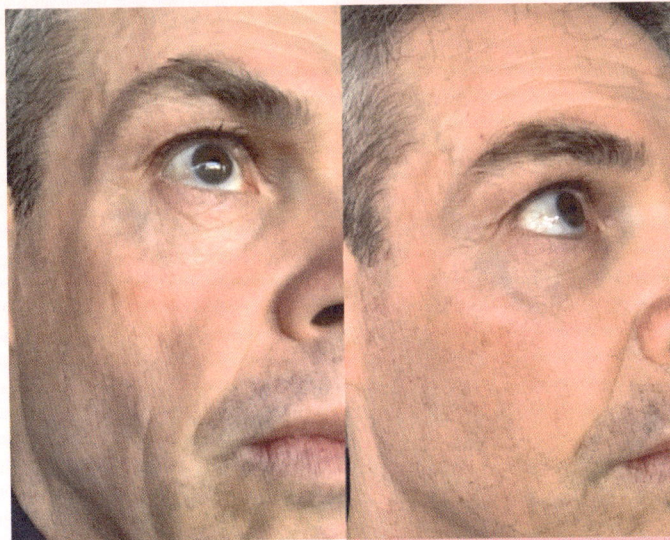

Day 1

Day 83

Individual results may vary.

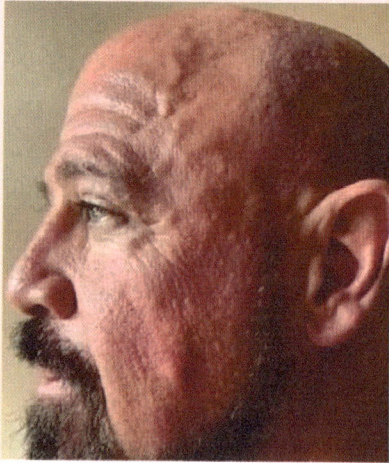
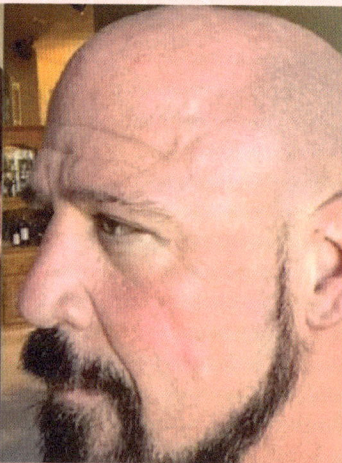

Day 1 | **Day 30**

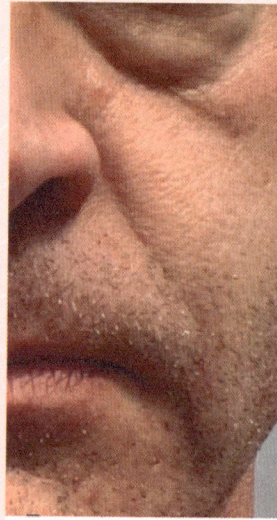
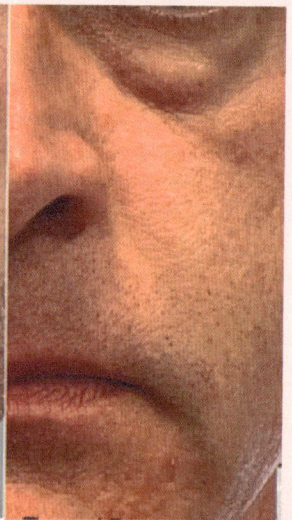

Day 1 | **Day 45**

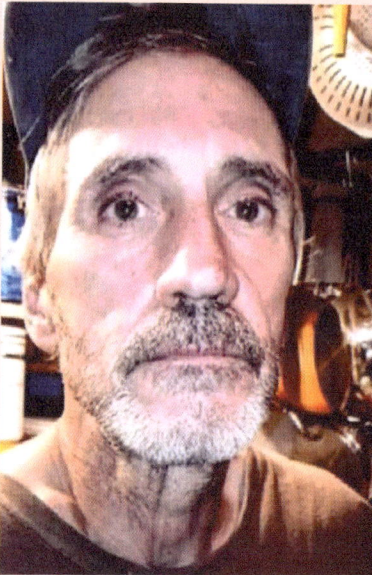
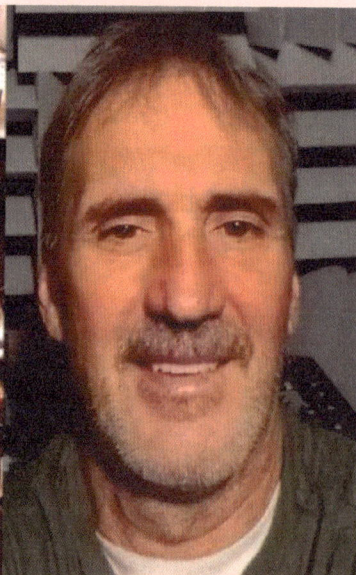

July 2021 | **July 2023**

Started on TriSynergizer and Axio, then introduced Collagen in 2022.

Individual results may vary.

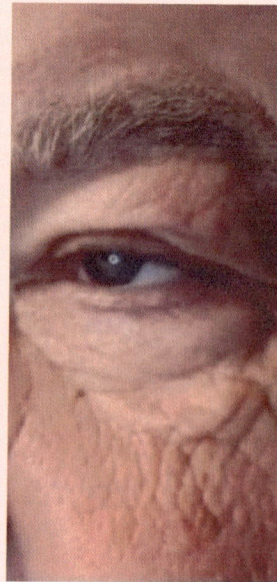
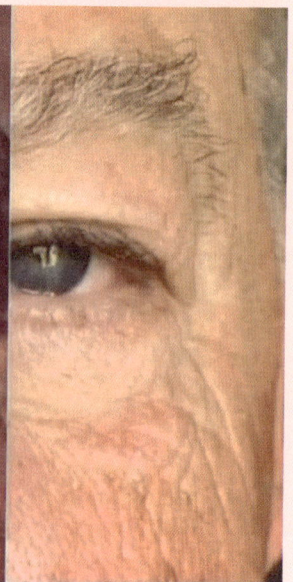

Before | **After**

for your hair, skin and nails

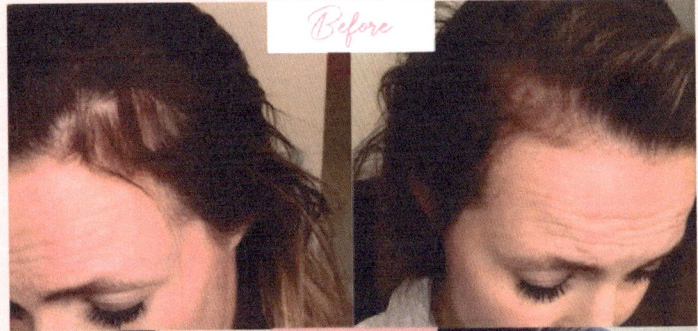

Before

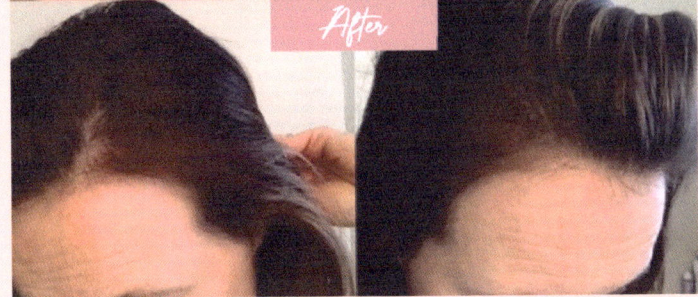

After

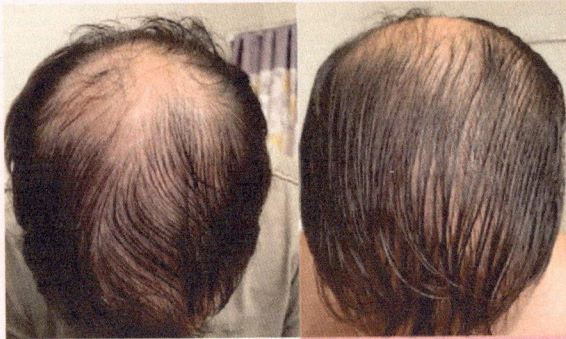

Day 1

Day 90

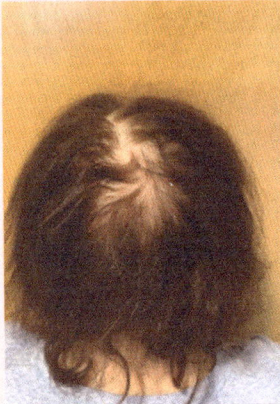

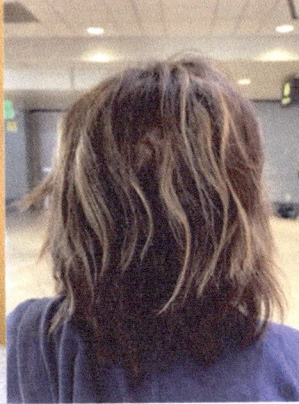

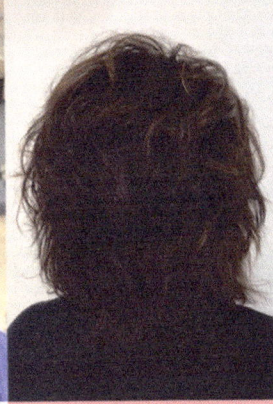

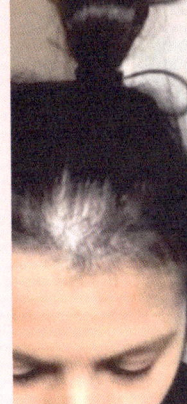

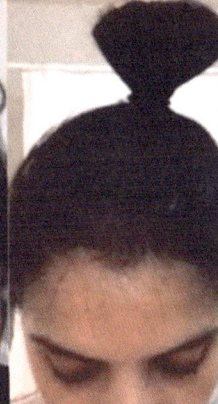

Early 2022

June 2022

April 2023

Before

After

Individual results may vary.

Benefits beyond great skin!

Nail health	Hair growth	Muscle recovery	Joint support	Gut health	Bone strength	Eye health
Liver detox	Cardio flexibility	Sleep quality	Mood support	Brain health	Cognitive support	Sexual support

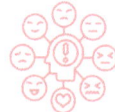

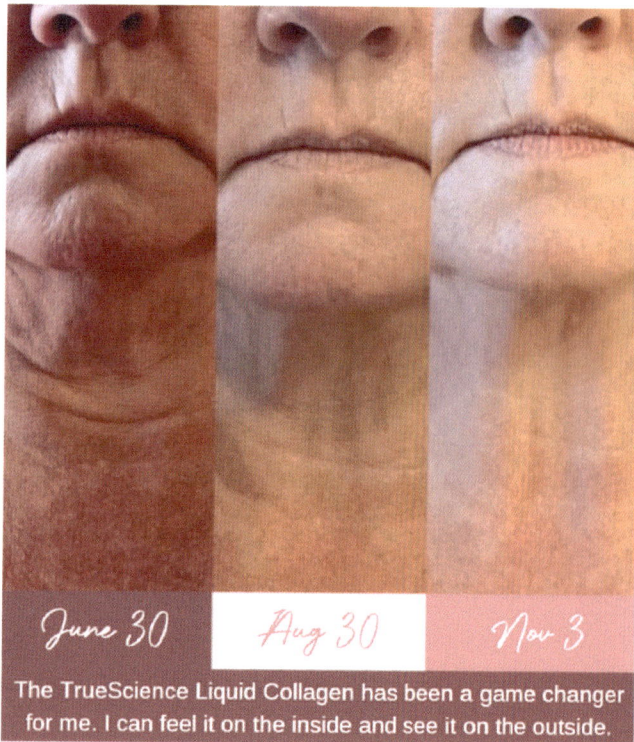

June 30   Aug 30   Nov 3

The TrueScience Liquid Collagen has been a game changer for me. I can feel it on the inside and see it on the outside.

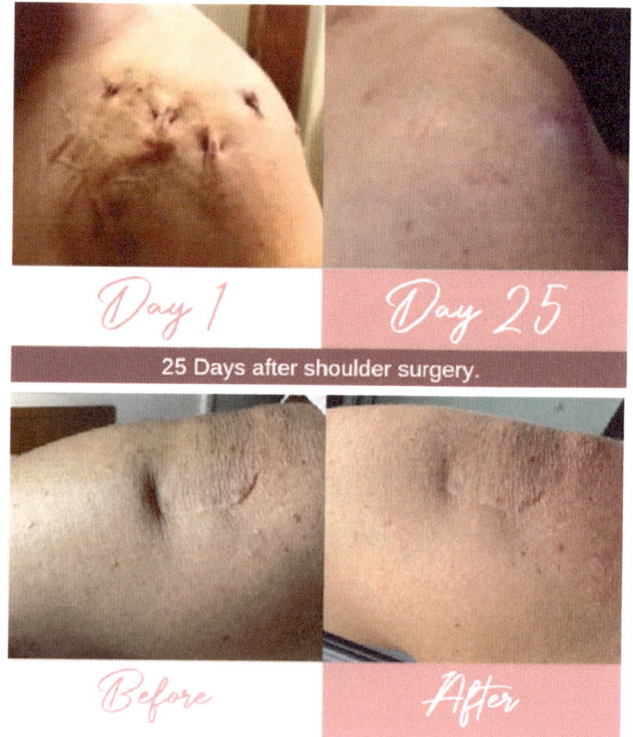

Individual results may vary.

Day 1   Day 25

25 Days after shoulder surgery.

Before   After

Day 1
Day 3
Day 5
Day 7
Day 10
Day 14

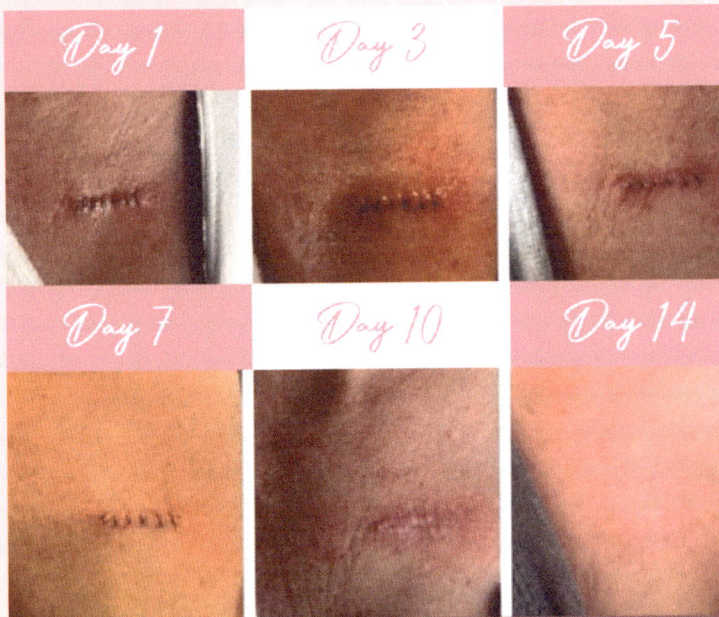

Nrf2 + Collagen following Basal Cell Carcinoma Removal.

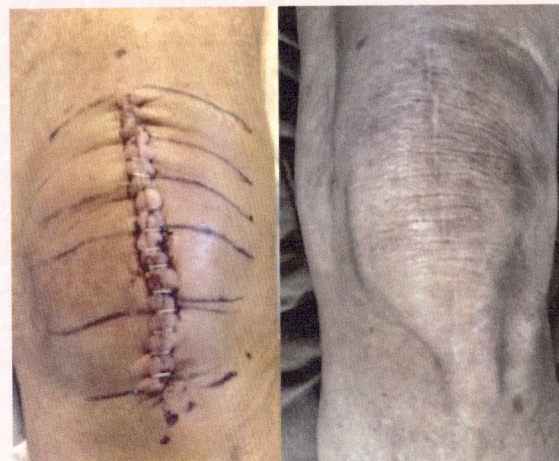

Day 1
2.5 Months

Mary Jo: "Split my kneecap in half! I used Nrf2 + TrueScience Collagen and in 2 1/2 months healed and barely noticeable."

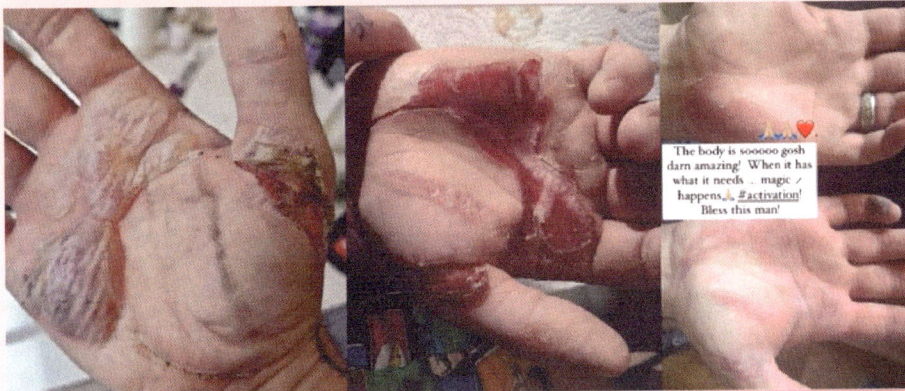

The body is sooooo gosh darn amazing! When it has what it needs .. magic happens. #activation! Bless this man!

May 22
May 27
June 10

3rd and 4th degree burns. 20 days on Activated Liquid Collagen and Nrf2.

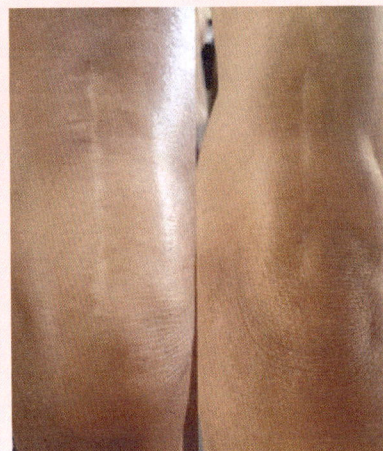

Day 1
Day 90

Individual results may vary.

Before | 3 weeks | 6 weeks

Nrf2, Omega, Collagen

Before | Day 7 | Day 13

Before | Day 14 | Day 30

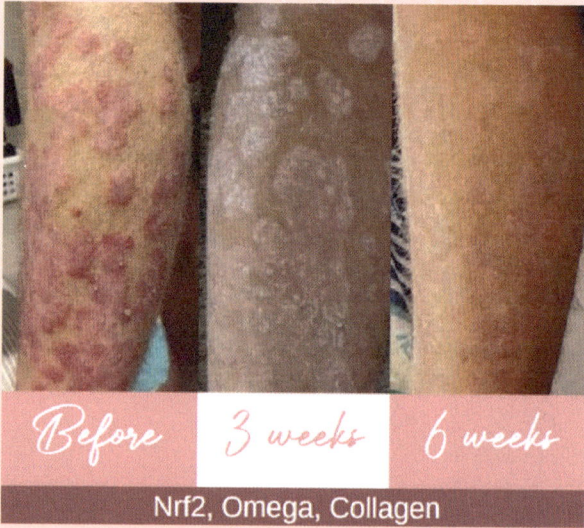

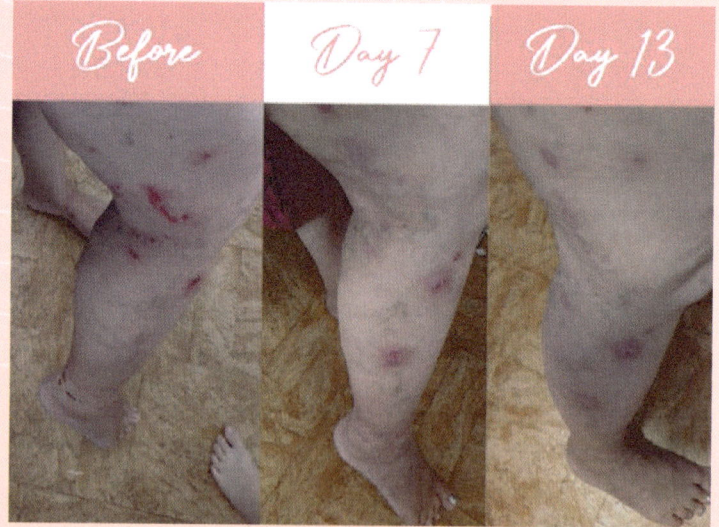

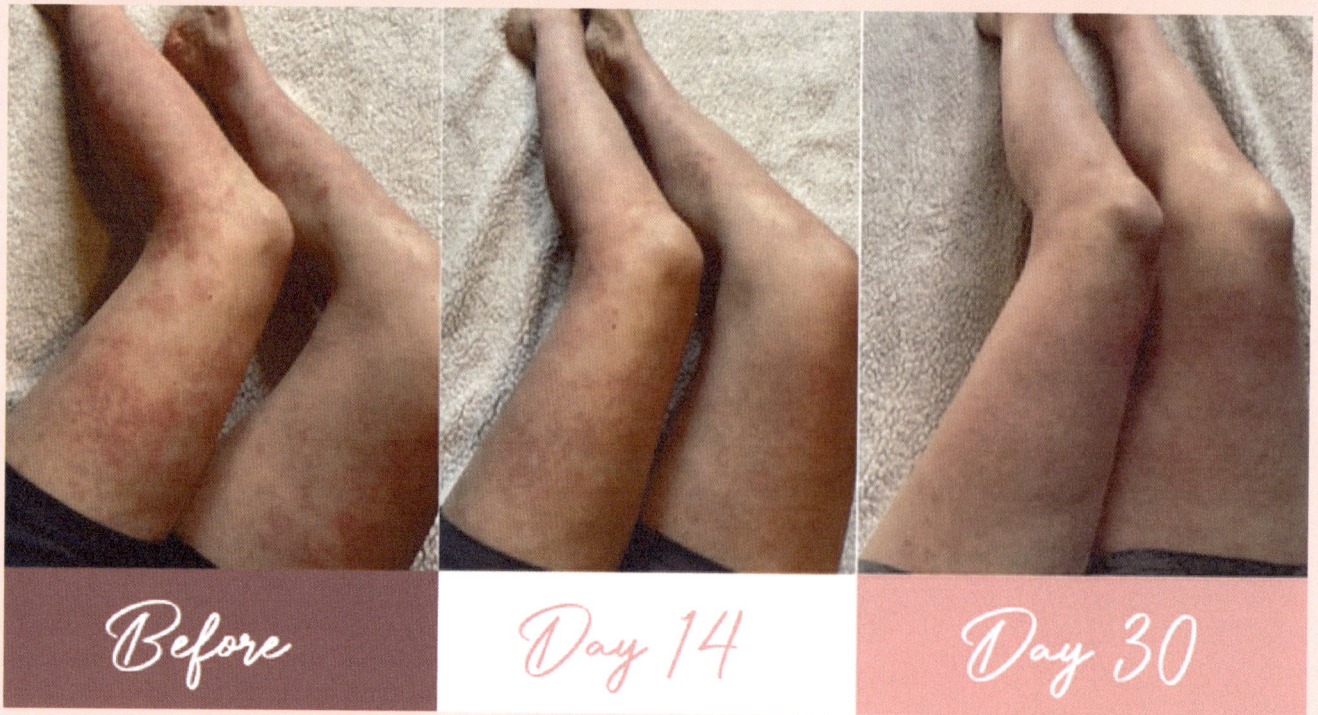

Individual results may vary.

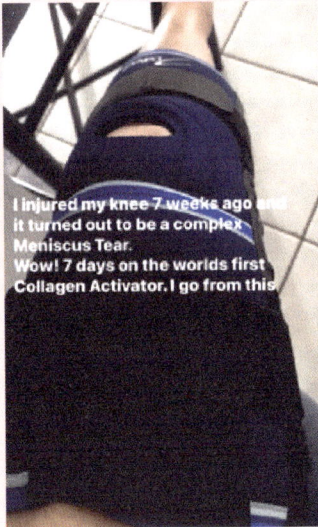
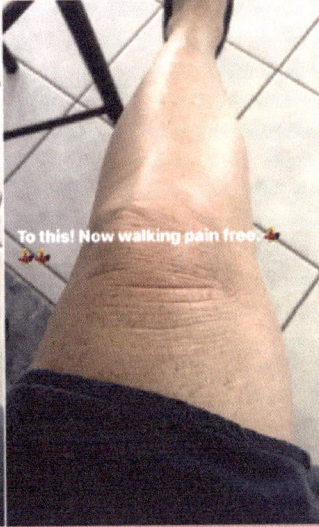

I injured my knee 7 weeks ago and it turned out to be a complex Meniscus Tear. Wow! 7 days on the worlds first Collagen Activator. I go from this

To this! Now walking pain free.

Day 1

Day 7

Meet my husband Terry. Even more important than the pictures.. Terry has gone from taking 4 extra strength Tylenol and 8 ibuprofen daily for RA pain to zero this week! 11 days on liquid collegen. Just incredible!

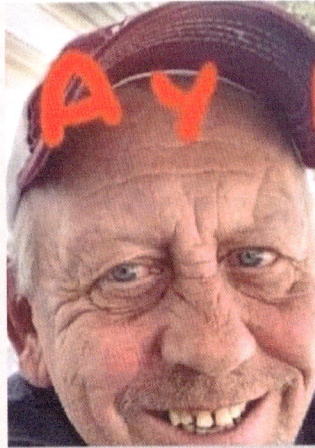
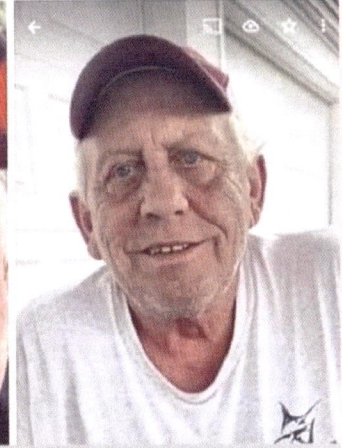

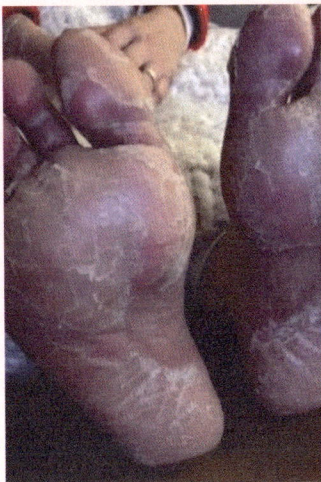
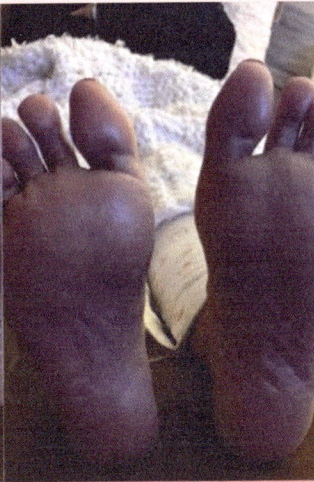

Before

After

Individual results may vary.

Hi Gillian just to let's you know all my blood test results is very good 👍 is better's than last one be for I take protandim NRF2. Hopefully 🤞 for next blood test even better and I no need take cholesterol tablets I only take 5 ml , the low dose but I like not takeking at all that the new from me have a good weekend 👍😍

Nrf2 + TS Liquid Collagen

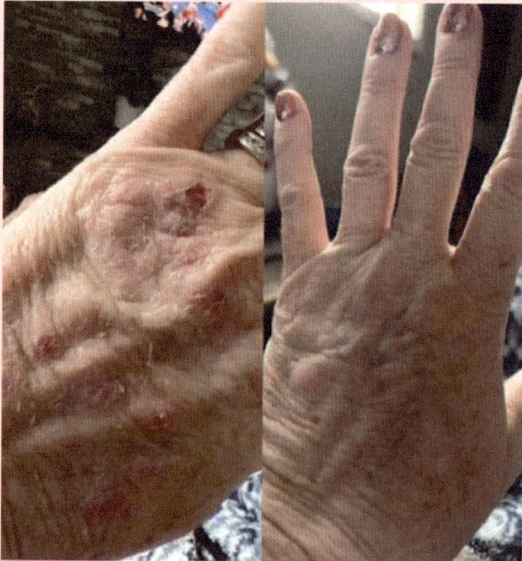

Before

After

It's pretty incredible! I'm actually still feeling, but the physical signs have gone away

Healing

Yeah, nothing was working so the collagen is definitely doing great work

Not to mention that my shoulder pain has been drastically reduced

What I forgot to put a picture of was not my arm I had a bunch of scabs on it that are now gone too

Good morning Gill. So I think the collagen is helping with my cramps. It is the only thing that I have changed in my life and instead of having an average of 3 cramps a night I have only had about 3 cramps in a week. I have been taking it in the morning with my other tablets. I have been taking it for nearly 2 months now. ☝️

❤️

I was taking it and stopped for some reason. Now my joints hurt and my feet are swelling up again. When I was taking it before my left foot and kankle was always swollen. It really took care of that. I'm going to get back on it!!

Bob
Others have told me that I am looking younger but that is not what I am excited about. Since being on the   Liquid Collagen, my knees do not hurt any more and more important my back is pain free. The Greatest Blessing, we have experienced in our home is that My Wife, B   no longer is experiencing the pain she has lived with for decades in her knees. What a Great Blessing!!!

Debbie
Oh definitely my joints! No soreness at all. No stiffness in my knees the next day after playing pickleball for 3 hours every Saturday and Sunday morning. 🤩

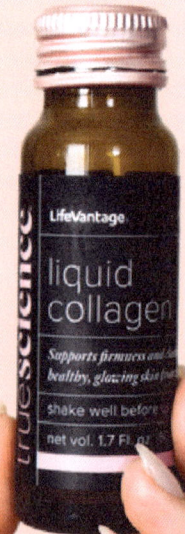

Ashley █████
Gut health has improved immensely! No more bloating. Always regular. Also hair is thicker and has a healthier shine to it. No more sparse hairline. Nails grow like crazy and are super strong. Skin and lips are less dry. Thicker lashes. 😊 Definitely worth the investment!

Individual results may vary.

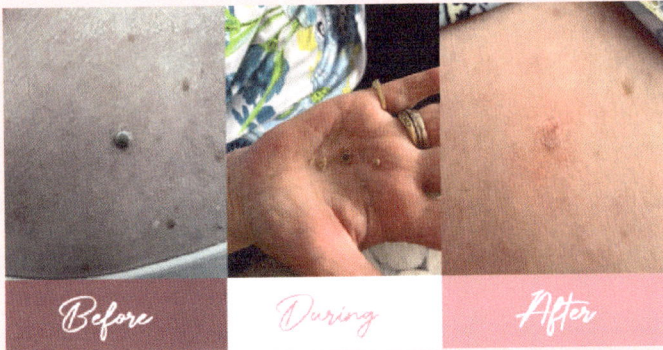

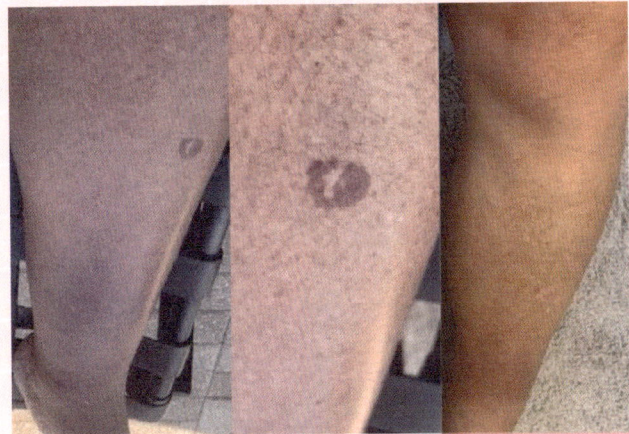

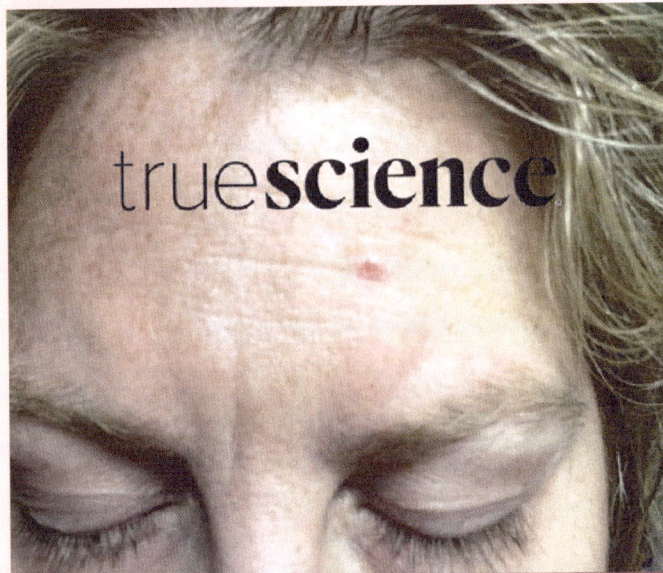

truescience

"My doctor would check out this mole/skin tag every year when I went for my annual physical. After 6 months on Activated Liquid Collagen, it is totally gone... literally fell off in 2 pieces like a scab."

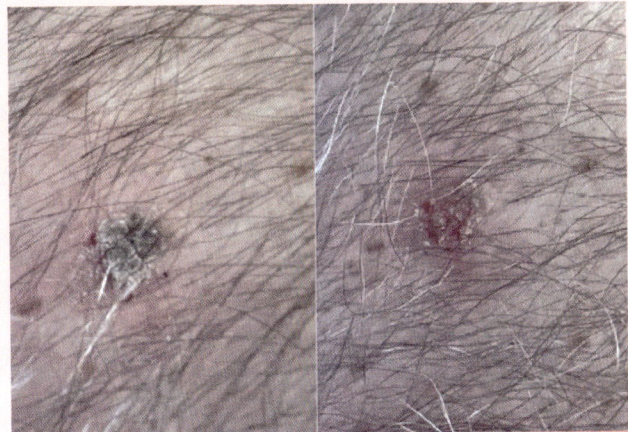

Aimee

"Good Morning! So this was a mole that has been on my forehead forever!! It came off over the weekend which I thought was just the top layer. Today I look and it's so smooth even though it's red! I really think it's gone finally!!!!!! This is so crazyyyyy!"

Activated with Nrf2 5 months
Activated Liquid Collagen 30 days
Activated Skincare System 90 Days

Individual results may vary.

consistency is key...

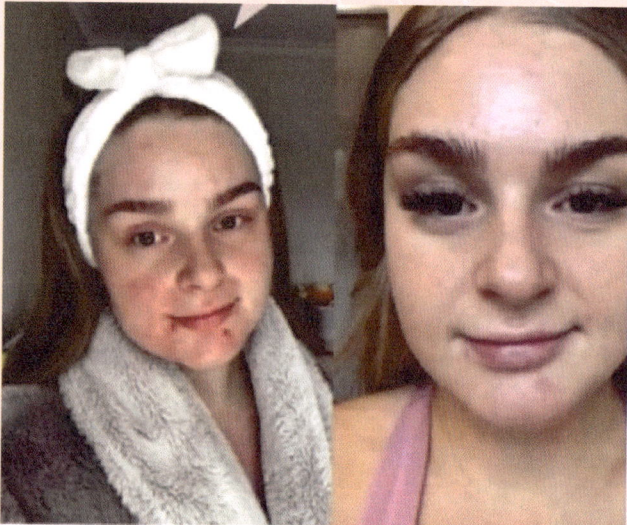

Day 0 | 2 Weeks

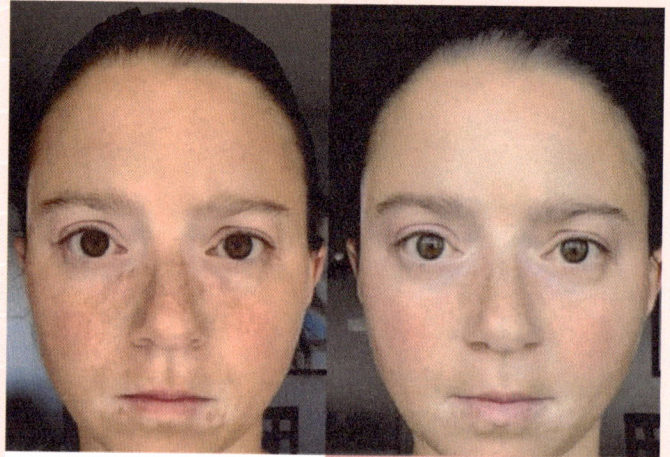

Day 1 | Month 5

Julie

"I was going to wait until tomorrow but I can't! I haven't done a side by side in a little bit and decided since it's been 5 months it was a good time. Well holy smokes I blew myself away! Isn't this true... people see things in and about us before we do? Or we may feel things inside our bodies but doubt if there is really change? I've been guilty of that for sure. Except the past 4 years have taught me A LOT about trust and intuition and belief.
So take a look for yourself. This is me 5 months apart. Sure my skin isn't as tan now but boy oh boy it is smoother. My sleeping is even better than it was. My dreams are vivid and I remember them! I am more balanced overall, my gut is happy happy!
PS Someone thought I was 22... Shhh I'll be 38 in January."

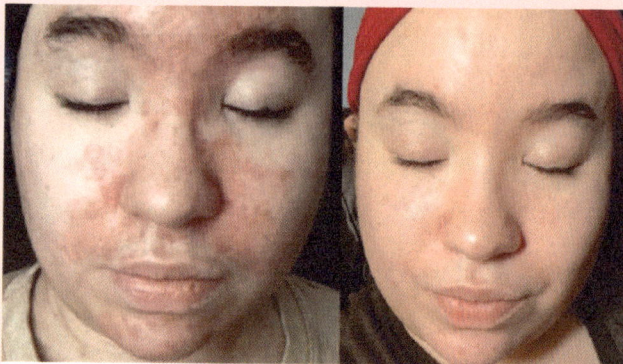

Day 1 | Day 14

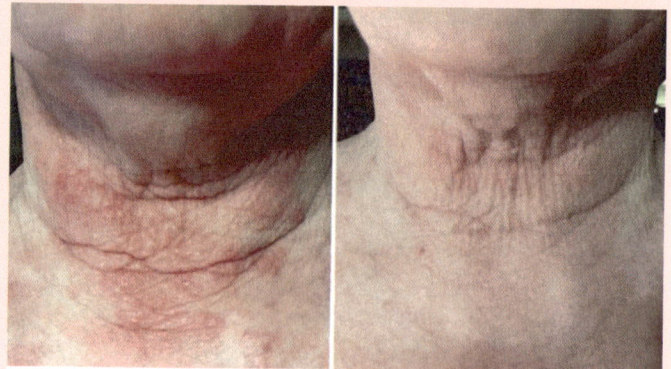

Day 1 | Day 50

Individual results may vary.

HOW DOES IT COMPARE?

liquid collagen *Comparison Chart*

	activates collagen*	replenishes collagen	maintains collagen**	collagen source	hydrolyzed	collagen amount	portable ready to drink	activates superoxide dismutase	Liquid bioavailable	price per serving	number of collagen strains
truescience® liquid collagen	✓	✓	✓	marine	✓	5,000mg	✓	✓	✓	$5.25	10
Nuskin Collagen+	✗	◑	✗	bovine	◑	2,500mg	◑	✗	◑	$4.13	?
Isagenix Collagen Elixir	✗	◑	✗	marine	◑	5,000mg	◑	✗	◑	$4.40	?
Tranont Glow	✗	◑	✗	bovine	◑	11,000mg	✗	✗	◑	$4.33	1
Modere Liquid BioCell Pure	✗	◑	✗	chicken	◑	<1,000mg	✗	✗	◑	$4.43	1
Modere Liquid Biocell Skin	✗	◑	✗	chicken	◑	<3,000mg	✗	✗	◑	$4.74	1
Younique DailyYou Shot	✗	◑	✗	marine	◑	5,000mg	◑	✗	◑	$3.30	?
YoungLiving Inner Beauty	✗	◑	✗	marine	◑	5,000mg	◑	✗	✗	$2.59	1
Vital Proteins Collagen Powder	✗	◑	✗	bovine	◑	20,000mg	✗	✗	✗	$1.80	1

*truescience® liquid collagen activates natural collagen synthesis by upregulating genes involved in skin barrier health, antioxidant production and collagen product TGM1, KRT1, KRT10 by 5x. SOD gene is activated 2700%. Catalase gene is activated up to 202%. COLA1A2 gene (type 1 collagen production) is increased by up to 42%.
**truescience® liquid collagen decreases the MMP9 gene by 33% which degrades and remodels collagen.

These statements have not been evaluated by the Food and Drug Administration. These products are not intended to diagnose, treat, cure or prevent any disease.

*activate. replenish. maintain.**

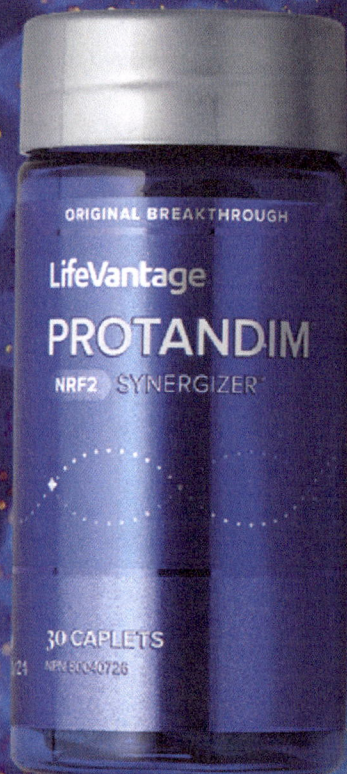

Protandim®
Nrf2 Synergizer™

reduce oxidative stress

*Support your body's own production of powerful antioxidants to fight the signs of aging.**

Dairy-Free Gluten-Free Vegetarian Halal Free from artificial colours, flavours, and sweetener

Oxidative Stress

If you are like 99% of the population... stressed out, sick, tired, and aging too fast - despite eating well, taking supplements and trying all the new fad solutions... chances are your Oxidative Stress levels are high.

But what causes Oxidative Stress??

Beyond BREATHING oxygen (yes, we create free radicals simply by existing) most of our oxidative stress comes from the taxing environment we live in.

EMF Radiation
Cell phones, tablets, laptops, WIFI, blue tower, 4G/5G/LTE, bluetooth, dirty electricity and more!

Chemical Exposure
Studies now show there are more than 80,000 (mostly untested) chemicals in our environment.

Psychological Stress
Triggers a cascade stress hormone and cytokines that break down cells and wreak havoc.

Poor Diet
GMO's, gluten, food dyes, preservatives, artificial sweeteners, seed oils, sugars and more!

Obesity
Causes a rise in particular hormones/adipokines that create low level cellular inflammation.

Sedentary Lifestyle
Is a risk factor for cardiovascular disease by damaging vascular function through OS.

Smoking + Alcohol
In addition smoking and vaping, secondhand smoke and alcohol consumption causes cellular damage.

Poor Sleep
Not only causes OS but high levels of inflammation impacts sleep quality.

Illness
Viral infections can cause a reduction in glutathione, impairing the ability to lower OS.

Early indications your body has high levels of oxidative stress:

- Poor Sleep
- Lack of Energy
- Headaches
- Aches and Pains
- Poor Immune system
- Stress and/or Moody
- Digestive Issues
- Depression and Anxiety
- Poor Attention, Focus and/or Brain Fog

Our body's natural ability to fight free radicals declines sharply with age and environmental factors.

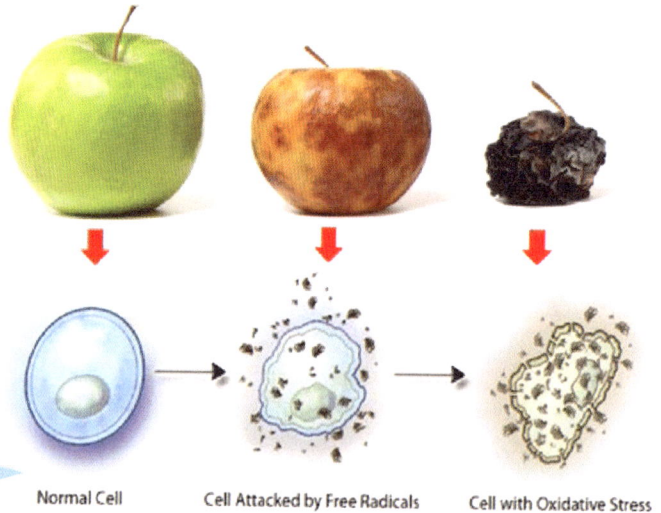

Normal Cell   Cell Attacked by Free Radicals   Cell with Oxidative Stress

WHAT HAVOC IS OXIDATIVE STRESS CAUSING IN YOUR BODY?

BRAIN
Alzheimer's, Parkinson's, MS, ALS, OCD, ADHD, Autism, Migraine, Insomnia, Depression, Dementia, Bi-Polar Disorder, Cancer

EYES
Macular Degeneration
Retinal Degeneration
Cateracts

HEART
Heart Attack, Stroke, High Blood Pressure, Atherosclerosis, Angina

LUNG
Asthma, COPD, Allergies, Chronic Bronchitis, Cancer

KIDNEY
Chronic Kidney Disease, Renal Nephritis

BLOOD VESSELS
Atherosclerosis, Hypertension Varicose Veins, Elevated Cholestrol and Triglycerides

SKIN
Wrinkles, Acne, Eczema, Psoriasis, Dermatitis, Cancer

IMMUNE SYSTEM
Chronic Inflamation, Auto-Immune Disorders, HIV, Herpes, Crohn's, Hepatitis, Colds & Flu, Lupus, Cancer

JOINTS
Rheumatoid Arthritis, Osteo-Arthritis, Psoriatic Arthritis

MULTI-ORGAN
Diabetes, Chronic Fatigue, Fibromyalgia, Heavy Metal Toxcity, Lyme Disease

This is just a partial list of conditions linked to high levels of oxidative stress. You can also search 'Oxidative Stress' + 'Your Condition' on pubmed.gov and see all the links. There are currently more than 300,000 studies on Oxidative Stress on Pubmed, the National Library of Medicine.

Protandim®
Nrf2 Synergizer™

Little Yellow Activator, the discovery that changed everything. It's one of the most groundbreaking insights into reducing oxidative stress, the cellular damage caused by free radicals. Oxidative stress is a key contributor to the signs of aging, and Protandim Nrf2 Synergizer is the only supplement shown to reduce oxidative stress by 40% in just 30 days. This finding is backed by over 30 independent studies conducted by institutions such as Harvard, Ohio State, and the American Journal of Physiology, among others.

How does it work? Your body produces its own antioxidants to fight free radicals, but production begins to decline in your early 20s. Protandim Nrf2 Synergizer activates pathways to support your body's ability to produce antioxidants, reduce cellular stress, and repair your own cells. It's a powerful, patented, all-natural solution to support your body's healthy aging process.*

Benefits:

- ◆ Reduces oxidative stress by 40% in just 30 days *
- ◆ Significantly reduces cellular stress through Nrf2 activation *
- ◆ Produces enzymes capable of neutralizing more than 1,000,000 free radicals *
- ◆ Supports the body's natural ability to repair and rejuvenate its own cells *
- ◆ Helps the body detoxify genes and regulate its survival genes
- ◆ Increased the median life span of male mice by 7%*
  (Source: National Institute on Aging)

*These statements have not been evaluated by the Food and Drug Administration.
This product is not intended to diagnose, treat, cure, or prevent and disease.

Green Tea
Green tea (Camellia sinensis) comes from the same native Asian plant as black tea called Camellia Sinensis. What makes green tea different, and green, is not the plant used to make the tea, but the way it is processed.

Turmeric Root
Turmeric (Curcuma longa) is a rhizomatous herbaceous perennial plant of the ginger family Zingiberaceae. Native to tropical South Asia, it needs temperatures between 20°C and 30°C, as well as a considerable amount of annual rainfall, to thrive.

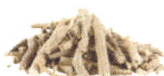

Ashwagandha
Ashwagandha (Withania somnifera) grows as a short shrub with a central stem from which branches extend radially in a star pattern. It is covered with a dense matte of wooly hairs. The flowers are small and green, while the ripe fruit is orange-red and has milk-coagulating properties.

Milk Thistle
The milk thistle (Silybum marianum) is a tall, flowering plant with spiny stems and toothed, thorny leaves. Even though it is native to the Mediterranean, this plant can be found throughout the world.

Bacopa
Bacopa (Bacopa monnieri) extract is taken from the succulent leaves of a small creeping plant commonly found growing throughout the damp and marshy wetlands of India. This herb, with its small white flowers, is often mistaken for a water lily since the 2 are related.

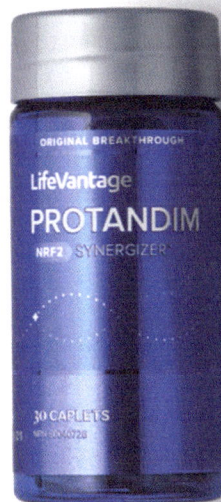

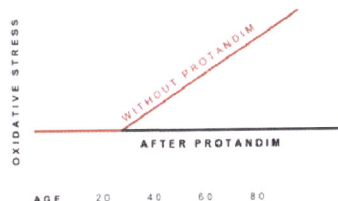

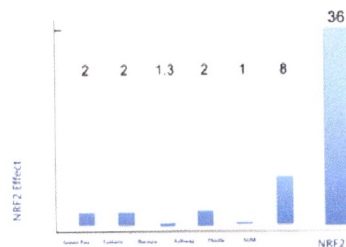

The Gift of Activation

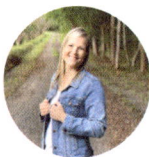

Join our Activate Wellness Facebook Community to see hundreds more success stories like these. Ask your Consultant to get you added.

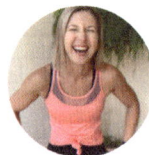

"These are just a few of the benefits within my family: Skin improvements, Weight gain and growth issues resolved after MANY years of searching for solutions, Gut health improvements, Energy and focus leading to better attention during lessons and higher achievements, Seasonal sniffles and sneezing reduced greatly, Brain Fog and Afternoon slumps disappeared, And SOOO much more!" Katie K

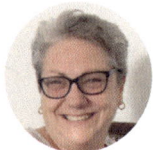

"I have suffered from a very unhealthy liver for years. I had tried everything before starting Nrf2. 8 months into activation I had new blood tests done. The Doctor was so impressed! All of my bloods were excellent, my liver and kidneys were the best he had seen in years." Denise H

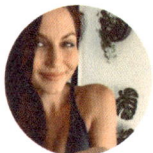

"For 8 months, I struggled with breathing difficulties, insomnia, fatigue, headaches, allergies, sore throat, an aching body, intestinal issues; extreme bloating & horrible PMS symptoms... the list went on. I got tested for every single disease & illness. (They were all clear!) I felt completely defeated. So I tried this golden activator & within weeks EVERY SINGLE SYMPTOM DISAPPEARED! I could literally feel every cell in my body being cleansed. I am now, alert/focused, energised, happy & extremely healthy!" Amy H

"3 years ago, I was suffering from migraines, headaches, sinus infections, no energy, brain fog, puffy, weight gain, anxiety, stressed, anemic, adrenal fatigue omg I didn't realise how sick I was until I started feeling better. Thank goodness for activation. I feel better than ever." Sarah VW

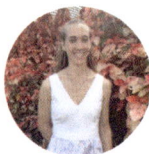

"I was introduced to Activation when I was working full time, my husband home with a back injury, and a 1 year old at home who was still feeding. I was exhausted and felt challenged trying to juggle everything. My health wasn't at its best and it was showing. A Mum in my class shared activation with me which I spent a lot of time looking into. I decided to give it a try and within a short time I was so glad to have my energy and passion for life back. " Ashleigh S

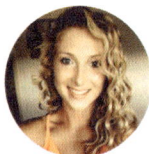

"As an exercise physiologist, I have always taken good care of myself, however, I was struggling with hormone health concerns that were causing havoc. I had tried many natural alternatives without success, but when I looked into the science of activation, I knew it was something I wanted to try. After 3 months, I had undeniable improvements and have been activated and healthy ever since." Sarah P

ACTIVATE WELLNESS

We do not make any claims to treat, prevent, cure or mitigate any disease or illness. Individual results may vary.

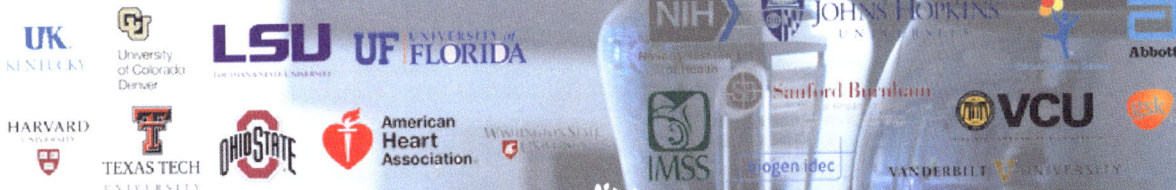

The perfect pair

LifeVantage's flagship product, Protandim NRF2 Synergizer has over 30 peer reviewed published studies, 7 patents, and is the only supplement proven to reduce oxidative stress (free radical damage) by 40% in 30 days.

Paired with our TrueScience Activated, hydrolyzed liquid collagen; this powerful combo is proven to increase collagen density by 100% and reduce unnecessary stress responses in your body. You will be feeling and looking your best from the inside out and outside in.

TrueScience® Liquid Collagen + Protandim® Nrf2 Synergizer™
100% Increase in Collagen Density

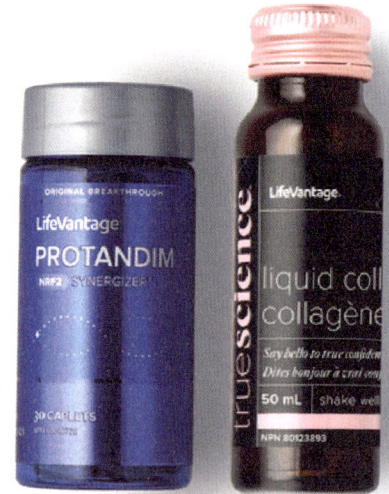

*Patented Combination

Help Fibroblast cells REDUCE unnecessary signaling, RECOVER from stress, and RESTORE optimal funtion.

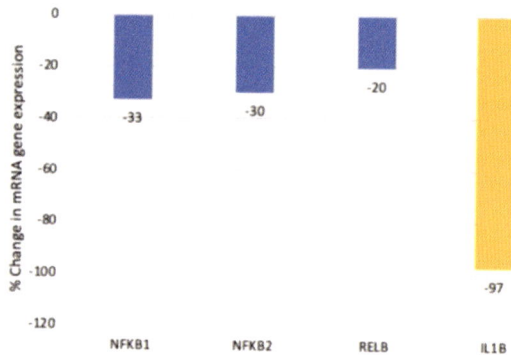

% Change in mRNA gene expression

NFKB1	NFKB2	RELB	IL1B
-33	-30	-20	-97

Less stress & breakdown = repair & rebuilding of collagen happens faster!!

For best results:

Take 1 Protandim Nrf2 Synergizer tablet and drink 1 bottle of Liquid Collagen per day.

Get Started! Get Results! Contact the person that shared this book with you:

30-Day Money Back Guarantee

Flexible Subscriptions

Printed in Dunstable, United Kingdom